IT IS MY EARNEST HOPE THE BOOK YOU HOLD WILL BRING

ORDER, OUT OF DISORDER

HOPE

INSPIRATION

TO OUR FELLOWS IN OUR WORLD OF PARKINSON'S DISEASE AND OTHER MOVEMENT DISORDERS

This book is dedicated to all who suffer with Parkinson's Disease or other Movement Disorder but will cast aside despair in their quest for a good and fulfilled future.

Edgar M. Nash
2800 Braden Ave., #35,
Modesto, CA 95356
edmnash@gmail.com
ed86_1920@sbcglobal.net

Dear Reader,

It is my most heartfelt wish all ParkinPeople who read this book will derive as much benefit from its contents as I have. In it are my research findings and personal discoveries, combined with whatever I have learned about life and living it during the 87 years of my earthly presence.

I am well into the progression of Parkinson's, and my observations regarding its effects on us and our attitude toward that plague are based upon truths extracted from personal experience and my acceptance of it as nothing worse than the equally irreversible and compounding effects of ageing.

Each day can be a treasure if we have meaningful and achievable goals. We cannot set a goal without expectation of success, a powerful factor that generates new energy found in our determination to go on with life and live it to the fullest.

I call it *"Positive Attitude"*.

Sincerely,

P>S> I will welcome your critique when you have read and know this book.

LIVING VERY WELL WITH PARKINSON'S DISEASE and other MOVEMENT DISORDERS

WE STILL CAN HAVE IT ALL!

If each of us honestly and thoroughly examines our latent skills and capabilities that live within, we will find an unused ability, skill or talent.

It is there! Recognize it! ***Use it!***

Possibilities are ***unlimited.***

In this ***encouraging*** book are many suggested GOALS and ideas for new careers, plus *original* ideas and positive directions *that really work* to assist my fellows in their quest for good living,

MY PARKINSON'S HAS GIVEN ME NEW DIRECTION IN LIFE THAT IS MORE REWARDING THAN BEFORE

LIFE IS GOOD

The following was copied word-for-word from the website of the United States Department of Health and Human Services. It tells us we are part of a extremely broad range of Americans: Coupling both those living with disabilities and our caregivers, we number more than:

100 MILLION!

THE NEW FREEDOM INITIATIVE

President Bush announced the NEW FREEDOM INITIATIVE on February 1, 2001, as part of a nationwide effort to remove barriers to community living for people with disabilities. Today, there are more than 54 million Americans living with a disability, representing a full 20 percent of the U.S. population. Almost half of these individuals have a severe disability affecting their ability to see, hear, walk or perform other basic functions of life. In addition, there are more than 25 million family caregivers and millions more who provide aid and assistance to people with disabilities.

SENSIBLE SELF-HELP FOR PARKINSON'S PROBLEMS

and

TREMOR, STROKE DISABILITY, TREMOR, PALSY, HUNTINGTON'S DISEASE, ATAXIA, DISABLED VETS, Etc.

ENLARGED PRINT EDITION

BY EDGAR M. NASH
Speaking from experience

Library of Congress Control No.2004098982

ISBN 0-615-12723-1

I invite suggestions for making this book more effective.
My e-mail addresses are:

ed86_1920@sbcglobal.net
and *edmnash@gmail.com*

website: ***www.edmnashbooks.com***

"*It is difficulties that show what men are".*
- Epictetus *(Discourses)*

This book is not for quitters.

It is for we who accept the consequences of ageing without question, and accommodate to Movement Disorders on the same terms. *We are thankful for the years already given, accept our condition in good grace and determined to attain a future of fulfillment!*

"*Mishaps are like knives, that either serve us or cut us, as we grasp them by the blade or the handle".*
- James Russell Lowell
(Fireside Travels)

Our book draws together and interweaves into its *encouraging!* fabric all the *essential* elements: Faith, Hope, Positive Attitude, Determination, Goals, Achievement and *Happiness!*

Although moving in harmony with doctors' instructions and treatments, this book *does not* provide medical guidance or direction, for I am not a doctor.

What it *does provide* is the OTHER HALF of complete treatment for Parkinson's and many other Movement Disorders by responding to the lack in conventional medicine of *practical psychological suggestion and application!* If each of us honestly and thoroughly examines our latent skills and capabilities within, we will find one or more unused abilities and aptitudes that will permit meaningful goals to be identified and achieved. That is the road to a future of good living!

* *Because Parkinson's Disease is one of the primary Movement Disorders, I will use either name in this text.*

In this book are never-before-printed descriptions of easily-applied and <u>*entirely original*</u> methods derived directly from my trial-and-error experiments that enable *releasing foot-freeze and easily initiating the first step*, *stopping hand tremor, easing swallowing, breathing and sleeping problems*, *setting attainable and meaningful goals*, and many other suggestions not only for improving our present condition but leading into a good future of true personal fulfillment.

At this writing in early 2008, medications and medical treatments currently in use are reported only as helpful information. But we can expect ongoing worldwide research will discover new medications and treatments that will make our lives ever easier, and eventually will overcome and defeat Parkinson's Disease and other Movement Disorders.

READERS SAY

"Mr. Nash demonstrates an insight into the coping strategies of Parkinson's Disease that are at times both simple and elegant. Upon reading his observations and discoveries, one realizes that his depth of thought is uniformly invested in all aspects of therapy."
Kevin O'Dell, M.D.
Neurology

To Edgar M. Nash -
"Thanks for sending your book, which we received. Your tips are very helpful - I learned from you. Thank you for putting the time and effort into this endeavor. I know many will benefit from your advice."
Susan Reese, Coordinator,
American Parkinson Disease Association
Midwest Regional Information and Referral Center, and
National Young-Onset Information and Referral Center.
1-800-223-9776.
www.youngparkinsons.org

Dear Mr. Nash,

Thank you for the opportunity to read and review your book. I am impressed with your text. You offer a lot of excellent information in a concise and detailed format. The most impressive thing is that the book is written from first-hand experience, not by a physician or researcher who has not been directly affected by Parkinson's.

This gives your book instant credibility. Most importantly, you go beyond providing clinical information by offering encouragement, motivation and hope.

The message I get from your book is to never give up. As a physical therapist, I tell my patients that every day is a blessing and it could always be worse. You have two choices in life: Give up or keep moving. The body is designed with the incredible ability to get stronger and exercise is the medicine that allows that to happen.

Again, thank you for the opportunity to review your book. It is an excellent resource for ParkinPeople and you should be proud of it.

God Bless -

Rob Mallory, PT

"Thank you for sharing your well-organized, information-filled and readable book on Parkinson's Disease with me, for I really enjoyed it. You certainly covered your subject matter in a very upbeat and complete manner."

Bettie Laird, MS, MSW

"Thank you for your new book – up close and personal with PD. It is a welcomed addition to our library."

Susan Reese, MA, RN, LCSW
American Parkinson Disease Association,
2100 Pfingsten Road, Room B100,
Glenview, IL 60026 (*www.youngparkinsons.org*)
847-657-5787 (*parkinsonscenter@enh.org*)
800-223-9776 (847-657-5708 Fax)

"Many thanks for your tips on Parkinson's. I am in the stage of shaking on the left side, especially my left hand, so those suggestions are perfect. My favorite chapter in your book is the one on attitude, and you do a good job not pushing God or Christ because you appeal to a wider audience so your readers can carry on with what they know."

Mrs. Lila Morgan, Honolulu, HI

"Your book is bound to help people with Parkinson's Disease who are tired of reading text-book style information about this sickness. Thank you for making it available."

Toni Hull, Marketing,
Epic Book Promotions,
594 Serrano Lane,
Chula Vista, CA 91910

"Hi, Ed,
As a nurse who works with Parkinson's patients everyday, I think Ed Nash's book is a work of encouragement and inspiration for patients because it comes from his personal experience."

Martha Godden, LVN
Clinical Nurse, The Parkinson's Institute,
1170 Morse Ave., Sunnyvale, CA 94089
(408) 734-2800 Main (408) 734-9208 Fax
www.parkinsonsinstitute.org
<http://www.parkinsonsinstitute.org>

OTHER BOOKS BY THIS AUTHOR

"COPING WITH MOVEMENT DISORDERS AND WINNING!" The only complete M.D. book that comfortably encourages a *positive attitude*, including *entirely original* directions not found elsewhere on how to cope with and ease the mental and physical problems associated with these terrifying illnesses. By an author who lives with Parkinson's Disease. Self-Published by the author.

"BINGO! BINGO! BINGO!" Boats Against Battleships. Guadalcanal, One December, 1942. A vivid World War Two story about PT boats during the intensive fighting for Guadalcanal and its vital Henderson Field ISBN 0970615795

"LOVE, SHAME AND GLORY" The World War Two Personal Wars of Edward Mason. Based on the author's own experiences during WWII, with several original and famous wartime photos. ISBN 0970615787

"PATENT YOUR IDEA YOURSELF . .WITHOUT AN ATTORNEY" and ***"SELF-HELP PATENTING FOR BROKE-FOLK"*** Complete instructions for the novice inventor to successfully obtain a utility patent.
ISBN 0970615752 and ISBN 0970615728

"WORLD WAR TWO USCG WARRIORS OF USS MENGES, DE 320" A complete history of the author's destroyer escort warship with a compilation of wartime histories of many of his shipmates. 2003. Self- published by the author.

"THE GREAT PINK TURKEY RACE" An illustrated children's book based upon an actual happening. Also ***"GRUNCHY-GROUCH AND THE HOLLYBERRY FAIRY"*** and ***"PEPPY PUPPY IN PARADISE"***. Illustrated children's books self-published by the author.

CONTENTS

Author's Statement 1
Dedication 2
Encouragement 3
The New Freedom Initiative 4
Title Page 5
This Book Is Not For Quitters 7
Reviews of This Book 9
Other Books by This Author 12
Contents 13
WE CAN WIN! 17

1 KEEP THE FAITH 25
Importance of Religion

2 WHAT'S THE DIAGNOSIS? 29
Is it a Movement Disorder?
Can it be NPH (Normal Pressure Hydrocephalus)?
Something else?

3 COPING WITH IT 31
Cut that barrier with *ATTITUDE*
Be thankful for the years already given
Short prayers that are meaningful

4 OVERVIEW 37
Adaptation, not despair!
Be positive!
What's detailed in this book and where

5 POSITIVE GUIDANCE
THAT REALLY WORKS! . . 41
How to initiate that first step
Walking for exercise
Walkers and wheelchairs
Hand tremor, relief of when: Seated, Standing, Walking, Lying down

Leg Tremor
Breathing easier
Sleeping better
Swallowing made easier
Speaking more clearly
Sitting and arising without problems

6 SETTING GOALS 65
Why it's so important
How to do it
Many choices

7 SPECIAL AND ENJOYABLE DIVERSIONS . . .73
Animal Pets
Birds and Fish
Flowers and Plants

8 SUPPORT GROUPS 77
How to locate your group
What to expect if you join
Internet support details

9 CAREGIVERS 81
Where to find your caregiver
Caregiver products and devices
Heimlich Maneuver described
Financial help for caregivers

10 MOVEMENT DISORDER RESOURCES 85
Help from Medicaid, Medicare
PD, other organizations listed,
E-mail and internet access
Assistive devices, sources of
Help for Children
Help for Women
Financial Assistance, sources described
Higher Education assistance
Housing assistance
Independent Living assistance

Legal rights described
Doctor Referral Services

11 EXERCISE 97
Why must we exercise regularly?
Health clubs
Exercising at home
Physical therapy facilities

12 DIET AND NUTRITION 111
Food and preparation suggestions
Vitamins

13 MEDICATIONS AND TREATMENTS . . . 113
Various Movement Disorders discussed
Many currently well-known Movement Disorder drugs listed
I.V. Glutathione for Parkinson's
Botox
Apokyn Physical Therapy

14 SURGERY 125
Activa Tremor Control Therapy
Pallidotomy
Thalamotomy
Deep Brain Stimulation
Gamma Knife Radiosurgery

15 ALTERNATE AND COMPLIMENTARY THERAPIES 129
Traditional Chinese Medicine
Ayurvedic Medicine
Herbal Medicine
Homeopathy
Relaxation, Meditation, Stress Reduction
Psychotherapy, Biofeedback
Prayer, Meditation, Guided Imagery
Laughter
Physical Therapy

Massage, Acupressure, Osteopathic, Reiki
Yoga, T'ai Chi, Naturopathy

16 SAVE ON DRUGS" PROGRAMS . . . 141
Several programs listed help people who cannot afford prescriptions

17 NUTRITIONAL AND HERBAL "SUPPLEMENTS" 143
Common vitamins and herbal items

18 COUNSELING 147
Why, when and how to arrange counseling

19 DRIVING 149
Cautions and suggestions
How to get around if not driving yourself

20 PERSONAL THOUGHTS 151
Closing remarks
Quotes from Irma Bombeck

21 WHAT WILL BE OUR LEGACY? . . 155

WE CAN WIN!

ARE WE BEING TESTED?

Whatever the *cause* of our condition, it is hugely important how we conduct ourselves following diagnosis, because it is at that point we are brought face-to-face with a major branch in the Road Of Life and a decision must be made. We have two, only two, choices:

1) We can give up and surrender to an enemy we could have fought and overcome.

2) We can *forgive* the cause, whatever it may be, *adopt a positive attitude* and move ahead into a good future of true accomplishment.

Although at the outset it may seem difficult, *we will adjust* and turn our attention inward to unused skills and abilities beckoning ahead, for untapped there lies the promise of personal fulfillment and contentment. It is a known fact that each of us has ONE OR MORE special abilities that, if recognized and applied, can and will provide direction into a fulfilling future

It truly lives there, and we can have it for the asking. But only if we live beyond mere hope, *and reach for it. Now think carefully . . . . .*

WHAT CAN I DO BEST?

When I contemplated that question in relation to my new condition and reluctantly acknowledging I no longer had all my abilities as before, I decided to proceed just as you will:

Go to Plan B, the thoughtful recognition of latent skills and abilities that will enable us to attain *GOALS* within reach, using the special abilities we always possessed but had not brought into regular use.

When we examine the embodiment of *goals* as such, we recognize each and every goal not as just a wish but as a *plan* to accomplish something *in the future.*

A whole chapter is devoted to SETTING GOALS, for when we do so we take a step ahead vital to elevating our sense of achievement and recognition of true progress, for from goal achievement springs pride of self and elevation of self-esteem.

HOPE is good and vitally necessary but it needs a *PLAN*, which by nature involves what we may call "directional discipline", for it provides direction of effort and requires discipline to effectively pursue and achieve our goals. If we are not already actively exercising our physical, mental and spiritual selves, but are willing to *help ourselves* improve and feel okay, we will find functional security in using the following contents to assist our putting together a Personal Plan and start the ball rolling.

At this point in Plan formation, it seems to me our Caregivers will become especially helpful in our identifying Goals that are sensible and important to us personally.

The order of distressful emotions listed below mirrors my own progress as I worked from initial diagnosis through successive *attitude* changes, and reflects what my studies show to be a typical evolution through the hurtful first stages of illness leading upward to <u>goal setting and achievement</u>. My own diagnosis of Parkinson's Disease immediately caused:

Angry Disbelief
Denial and Mental Isolation*
Depression*
An Awakening
Hope
Positive Attitude
Acceptance
Goal setting (Determination)
Achievement (Increased self-esteem)
Emotional Stability
Satisfaction

* *I was unwilling to communicate.*

Does that list look familiar?

In the list above, *Achievement* is the pinnacle, from which *Emotional Stability* and a strong sense of Personal Fulfillment assuredly will evolve. I firmly believe this book can and will assist your progress into your own Very Personal Victory through *achievement of meaningful goals.* My own experience has made me appreciate the importance of goals, for they keep me busy in all personal dimensions (leaving no room to feel sorry for myself!) and focusing always ahead on progress and achievement.

This book was my primary goal. My next goal will take about three months using my computer to scan, one-at-a-time, and print onto sheets of photo-grade paper hundreds and hundreds of ageing and fading family photos. *("Yes, Dear. I'll start right away, but why such a huge bunch of relatives? Let's whittle down your side of the family by ignoring the ones they hanged. OUCH!")*.

Additionally, I have a list of long-delayed but meaningful goals that may keep me busy the rest of my life, and I really look forward to digging into them, one at a time starting at the top. As the saying goes: Working on them will keep me busy, off the street, and out of trouble. . . . . *Sigh*

Think of all those attainable jobs you have backed up and list them in order of importance. Smile, pop your knuckles and get going now, *because you are looking at a future of interesting occupation*. But beware the consequences of success: Lazy distant relatives will hear about your determined penetration into the old and forgotten family historical treasury, and quickly will find their way to you with a deluge of neglected but suddenly urgent jobs. Don't open the door!

With the love and helpful constancy of the beautiful person to whom I am so very fortunate to be wed, I gradually but finally had come to discipline myself into acceptance of an unchangeable condition and move ahead into that part of my future *within my control,*. I had difficulty walking, and tremor began in my right hand, so I decided to experiment with new methods that had a chance to make such problems more bearable.

When I had made several new discoveries that greatly helped my walking (especially taking the first step easily), hand tremor, swallowing and other features with true promise to make my life better, I felt compelled to make them available to other people. To these ideas and suggestions I have added a treasury of factual and informative material taken from my research, and this book is the result.

This is a sensible guidebook organized to *materially* assist anyone with a Movement Disorder, while encouraging them *to toss aside despair and defeat, and adopt a positive attitude.*

The text is written in enlarged, easy-to-read 14-point type and phrased in an easily-understood manner as it describes and details facts, factors and features *practical* and valuable to all readers who seek support and encouraging guidance. All its provisions are intended to work in harmony with and to strongly fortify our physicians' directions, diagnoses and treatments.

In doing so it DOES NOT mirror the confusing and depressing medical-college-textbook writings of other Movement Disorder books and publications that magnify readers' agony by providing only depressing *medical and technical information.*

Although many thousands of books and other publications are out there, not a single, solitary one contains the simple yet very practical assistance to movement disorders described in this book, solutions that directly relate to those ever-present problems we face.

Why, for example, for those who have hand tremor strong enough to cause spillage from a drinking vessel, hasn't anyone else suggested simply holding that cup in the palm with our thumb through the handle, or glass in our upturned hand and drinking while steadying it with the other hand, if necessary?

The reason why that is so effective is detailed in Chapter 5: *"Positive Guidance That Really Works"*, which addresses easing hand tremor, initiating the first step, walking features, turning safely, relief of swallowing and breathing impairment, speech and writing improvement, and much other useful information. Also, the chapter on *Exercise* is very important, for mind and body are inter-dependent. *We all know the mind works best when the body is in good condition.*

We all may not acknowledge it, but we are *spiritual* beings. True comfort cannot be realized without having regular and frequent association with the transcendental power and life force we must acknowledge exists in everything and everyone. We may take the time to pray or attend religious services on an ongoing and daily basis so we can connect with our spiritual nature, but to neglect such a conscious union can be dangerous. For, if we are treated only in the physical sense, and neglect our emotional, psychological and spiritual selves, we not only are ignoring *complete treatment* of our condition but may be overlooking the most important elements in the retention or regaining optimum health and well-being.

1 - KEEP THE FAITH

I realize some of you may not be religious, but even so I sincerely ask that you walk with me through this page because *you may find additional strength and determination in it, a power beyond your pre-perceived limit that will renew and strengthen your inner self on a regular day-to-day basis.*

History tells us all peoples, all the way back into their earliest beginnings have identified and worshipped a single all-powerful ethereal force, even though some may have had many lesser deities that answer to a peak authority, each having specific power over some aspect of life. They worshipped in many ways, even by sacrificing human beings, but always and ultimately to the image of a supreme god-figure. Theirs was religious belief, however it may be construed, as are any and all of the devotions and creeds of today, all over this planet.

Sometimes, although we may have a deep and abiding belief in Almighty Providence, we may be drawn aside by disturbing influences and events, and come to question His omniscience. However, we can be assured by going outdoors on a clear night and looking upward, UPWARD . . . . .

Into the birthplace of Truth and Peace and Purity and Time, and be drawn into a gigantic symphony beyond any reckoning of depth and distance, glorious beyond thought and flashing with bright jewels set into the infinite universe to its furthest reaches, where myriads of stars and galaxies and planets and heavenly avalanches of beauty slowly cascade into a horizon of deep purple velvet as the mighty wheel of night slowly turns its limitless reaches of splendor.

How can we deny or doubt the power of His presence, when we are seeing into His very existence?

My most inspirational experience with prayer came to me in 1943 after two years of enlisted service in the U. S. Coast Guard during early World War Two in the South Pacific (that *really* dates me), when I was sent to Officers' Candidate School at the Coast Guard Academy in New London, Connecticut, for four months of intensive training to become an officer and (hopefully) a gentleman. On my first Sunday I attended Chapel.

The final part of the service was a wonderfully deep and rolling chorus as hundreds of strong men sang "The Sailors' Hymn", a seagoing man's most profound entreaty to his Maker, a powerful supplication set to stirring music I hadn't known of before.

Here are the inspiring words of the first three stanzas:

Eternal Father strong to save
Whose arm hath bound the restless wave,
Who bidd'st the mighty ocean deep
Its own appointed limits keep;
Oh, hear us as we cry to Thee,
For those in peril on the sea.

Oh Christ! Whose voice the waters heard
And hushed their raging at Thy word,
Who walk'st on the foaming deep,
And calm amidst its rage did sleep;
Oh, hear us as we cry to Thee,
For those in peril on the sea.

Most Holy Spirit! Who did'st brood
Upon the chaos dark and rude,
And bid its angry tumult cease,
And give, for wild confusion peace;
Oh, hear us as we cry to Thee
For those in peril on the sea.

2 – WHAT'S THE DIAGNOSIS?

Treatment for all Movement Disorders depends on the underlying cause, with the goal of the treatments being to relieve symptoms. Treatment may include medication, botulinum toxin (BOTOX) injection therapy, and surgery. *(Why doesn't this standard list include attitude improvement, goal setting and other powerful and effective therapies described in this book?).*

What if your diagnosis is wrong? What if you are being treated for symptoms of one Movement Disorder when you have another from which you may recover after proper treatment?

For example, physicians who specialize in diagnosis and treatment of Essential Tremor (ET) have reported one in three of their patients who came to them with previous diagnoses of ET actually were suffering with a different MD. Apparently the reasons for their mis-diagnoses were due to "overlapping" symptoms common to ET but also evident in Parkinson's Disease, Cervical Dystonia with Dystonic Tremor, Parkinson's Disease with Essential Tremor, and others that were misread and thought to conform with the true symptoms of ET.

Mis-diagnoses of ET apparently may occur when the patient reports early symptoms involving: (1) Only one arm or leg, or (2) A rest tremor, usually combined with a postural or kinetic tremor, or (3)

Dystonic posture, or (4) Slow, rapidly alternating movements, and (5) Decreased facial expressions.

There are other diseases that have some (or all) the symptoms as Parkinson's and other Movement Disorders, such as problems with gait or walking, with thinking, with bladder control. One is *"Normal Pressure Hydrocephalus"* (NPH) a condition caused by excess fluid exerting pressure on the brain. It pushes the brain outward and stretches the nerve fibers so they cannot function properly.

NPH is identified by an MRI: Magnetic Resonance Imaging Scan. This is an expensive procedure, but it can save the mis-diagnosed patient from future stress and heartaches. If you and your family have detected the three classic signs of NPH *(gait is worsening, thought processes are becoming less clear, and urinary incontinence)* you should insist on seeing a specialist in normal-pressure hydrocephalus and having a scan.

Treatment for NPH is a 45-minute procedure during which neurosurgeons surgically insert a tube called a shunt into the brain to drain excess fluid (up to 10 times the normal) and move it to the belly for absorption. Adjustments are made in the doctor's office with a magnet.

3 – COPING WITH IT!

When you were diagnosed with a MD, did you sense being suddenly encircled by an impenetrable barrier that seemed to overwhelm and possess you to the point of hopelessness with no escape? I will admit I was – at first.

The defense that will cut right through that wall is *attitude*. *POSITIVE* ATTITUDE.

Our positive determination to go on with life and make the most of it is set in motion and advanced *by accommodating to our condition,* a mindset that will defeat any and all negatives as we adopt and apply the many available assistive and helpful methods, means and devices of all kinds. There are many such choices printed on the pages to follow that can help make our futures bright and hopeful.

At the outset, *depression* usually follows in lock-step with the diagnosis of any serious Movement Disorder. Isn't depression a companion of despair? However, we know for a fact that despair can be replaced by *hope* when hope is generated by *determination* to maintain good health and mental attitude through the several avenues of well-being attainable by healthful physical and mental exercise, proper nutrition, goal-striving, association with people we love and respect, doing relaxing things we enjoy, and taking advantage of the therapies beneficial to PD patients.

When we are physically fit we have long known our mental self will function better, for the two are inter-dependent and work in harmony. When this happy state is present, our attitudes must by definition be elevated, for all our capabilities are enabled and we are assured of realizing our planned undertakings and goals.

One of the best medicines of all that doesn't cost a nickle, is *laughter!* We all acknowledge the enjoyment derived from a good laugh, and the feeling of lightness and comfort it brings. Sources of merriment are many, beginning with the company of people you like, and with whom you can carry on a lively discussion, trade funny stories and describe humorous events and family happenings.

Why not start a catalog of jokes that make you laugh that you can publish and give to others (a good way to make new friends).

Books can bring howls of fun, as can the right movies or TV programs. Will you list all that appeal to you? Will you act on that list, with the primary choice given priority? There's a Goal here - one you truly will enjoy. When you discuss this with your caregiver and others, there surely will be laughter!

Cooking can bring not only good times but an honest feeling of accomplishment, when we labor and bring forth a dish or complete meal that others enjoy and compliment.

My finest cooking triumph comes with a good beef steak marinated with (forgive me?) "*El Rancho Nasho* Teriyaki Sauce". Until you have tried it you *will not believe* how extremely good this steak will taste, especially when cooked over charcoal. For best results, try to get an imported Japanese *plain* soy sauce (some domestic soy such as Kikkoman is okay, although it is thinned with water).

Prepare the marinade by adding some fine-ground black pepper to a suitable puddle of soy in a platter, then a generous shake or two of garlic powder and a liberal dash of powdered ginger. Some daring folks may wish to add a wee bitty taste of cooking sherry (it won't blow up!). Mix the powders well into the marinade, then baste both sides of the meat with it and let soak thirty minutes before placing this masterpiece carefully and lovingly on the barbecue. Then don't let it out of your sight, or this will happen (Don't say I didn't warn y'all):

Upward and outward the aroma will soar
And quickly neighbors all a-rounding
On all your doors will be pounding
So prepare your defenses
For they'll jump over your fences
To devour the steak you adore

My recipes are much better than my "poetry", so please don't give up for here is another winner. If you like lamb chops, treat yourself to an unbelievably tasty treat of Teriyaki Lamb Chops, delicately cooked over charcoal and served with brown rice and a super salad or green veggie. Chicken skinned and de-fatted before marinating will cackle merrily with this loving treatment.

High-quality hamburger steak will prove unusually happy if brushed with this marvel of *haute cuisine exceptionale* before being popped over the coals, especially if the meat is laced with chopped fresh onion and served up with toasted slices of real sour-dough bread nicely smothered in melted extra-sharp cheddar cheese harmonizing with gobs of good baked beans! And a *salade supreme* set off with small apple chunks offering a special harmony with pretty little wrinkled-red tasty cranberry "raisins" singing the soprano part.

If your dinner companions like this sort of fare and are treated to it just once, they will positively drool when you even mention it again. This may result in your repeatedly being coerced into considerable extra effort to satisfy their craving. You may be forced into opening your own restaurant!

How about an "attitude-adjustment time"? Coffee hour, tea time, cocoa time, cocktail hour, music hour, etc., etc. are enjoyable when shared with others.

If a cocktail is of interest, try a (here we go again) "Special *El Rancho Nasho* Manhattan" made with a good and lovingly-aged "bonded" USA Bourbon whiskey (Kentucky?) shaken with a fine imported Italian *sweet* Vermouth (Cinzano?). Try one ounce of Vermouth to two of Bourbon, or adjust to taste, (and don't shake too much or you'll bruise the Bourbon or the ice. Or both) made really tasty by adding a Maraschino Cherry and a half-teaspoon of its juice *(that's important!)*. A small strip of crisp orange peel squeezed into the drink is very nice, too, and shows how very classy you are.

If you really, really want to show lots and lots of class, listen up. Cut a sizeable strip of *crisp* peel from a citrus fruit (lemon preferred for this masterpiece) and pinch a spray of the oil from the peel through a lighted match flame held right over a martini. There will be flaring as the oil spray zips through the flame, and you will see on the surface of the cocktail a speckling of tiny blackish dots, which are singed oil particles. This will change the flavor of the cocktail, which most folks consider to be upward. A martini loves this treatment, but the usual green olive hates it because it will be on the outside looking in, especially if its core is stuffed with little anchovy fishies.

Most people find comfort and inner peace in religion. However, even if non-religious you may find comfort in a place of worship while meditating in prayer or just sitting quietly and experiencing the power of His presence, letting it flow into you.

And listening.

Regular prayer is powerful therapy. It will help greatly in effecting and strengthening general "attitude adjustment". Attending church with a companion you like and enjoy can be especially rewarding. How about coffee and a muffin after the service? Join the choir! Your average voice is okay, and you do not have to sing like an angel. My injured daughter sang in the teenage choir sitting in a wheelchair. No sweat.

Photography can be the essence of satisfaction and a never-ending source of study and increasing ability without requiring much expense. I bought an excellent new camera on the internet, that serves up exceedingly fine imaging definition and even has close-in zooming ability, for just

$45.00. This is an easy vocation to get into, and there are photography clubs and groups that travel to nearby destinations offering interesting subjects. These people welcome newcomers, and if you don't drive will take you along as a passenger. And, there always will be someone with exceptional knowledge who gladly will take you on as a student.

Can you think of others? How about relaxing with music we enjoy and feel deeply, or organizing a group for regular round-robin tea-and-bridge parties (perhaps another game, or a complicated jigsaw puzzle) with people whose company you enjoy? Make a list (could be your first goal) and your eyes will brighten with fun ideas!

Don't overlook recorded books on tape or a CD. Don't have to do the reading. Just sit and enjoy while a gifted reader entertains you and your guests (from the Support Group?).

And then there's Mother Nature in all her resplendence, always there in her countless forms for your enjoyment. Here is a glorious subject for your photographic ventures.

4 – OVERVIEW

Ours are conditions that demand
adaptation,
***not* despair**

and can be kept in abeyance for many fruitful years, permitting us to live good, productive and happy lives, particularly if our attitude is kept *positive*..

We have the power to choose our own attitude. Isn't it the *POWER of our attitude* that determines changes in our condition, either negative or positive? A positive, determined-to-succeed attitude will strengthen the voice, straighten the back, power the step and put sparkle back into our eyes.

Those of us with a healthy determination to cope with our condition will develop high self-esteem arising from knowing true accomplishment, coupled with energy to persevere and pursue activities and relationships that give life real meaning. If we promise ourselves that much, we'll live meaningful lives.

NEVER GIVE UP! *NEVER!*

It is intended this book will provide readers a source of *simple, yet practical and useful* information that will prove to be the basis for better, happier living. *(If you think* ***we're*** *disadvantaged, just look around at so many other people, especially* *disabled firemen, police, and military warriors who live amiably with conditions considerably more disabling than ours).*

Contentment can be found when we accept our lot and proceed with vigor to look and *plan ahead* and make a good future happen by accomplishing with determination the factors of *self-help* set forth in this book. Maintaining a positive, upbeat attitude <u>will materially affect</u> <u>health</u>, even though at the outset of our diagnoses it may have been difficult to believe.

When you achieve a goal, brighten up *and give yourself a reward.* When your efforts seem temporarily futile, relax, forgive yourself and re-aim at your target goal so you can regain sense of control. Focus on small victories, one at a time, and continue with your determined efforts. Several small victories add up to a big win.

Little things do add up. Anything big cannot be big without containing many little things, can it? Doesn't that apply to us, and what we have learned we must do to have a good day? Let's combine all the little things we know are helpful to us into a wonderfully meaningful whole, filled with ideas to use and habits we have acquired that, when mixed with positives and a liberal dash of hope, will give us good living. All we have to do is let it!

Why not keep a journal of your daily experiences to chronicle your efforts, your achievements and your ongoing planning? Will it help others if published?

This book is not only directed to Movement Disorder patients, but to their Caregivers, those kind, beautiful and considerate persons whom I hope also will find benefit in these pages. Caregivers are necessary to us, and much is said in the chapter devoted to these blessed people, including suggestions regarding how and where to find (and receive) financial assistance for them.

In Chapter 9 is information relating where and under what conditions our non-professional caregivers are able to receive substantial financial compensation for their helping hands (more on this later). Most of such fine folk are spouses, family members, or other people dear to us.

We begin with the assumption neurologists or other physicians will have diagnosed your condition and prescribed medication(s) for treatment. And, almost surely, they will have laid down the law on some or all the self-help elements covered in this book, but we'll look at all sensible solutions that will act to fortify your determination to proceed into a future that holds promise of better living.

See in the chapter on *Medications and Treatments* for information not only on prescriptive drugs but some newer treatments that are not yet well-known but hold great promise. You will read about *Savings on Drugs*, too

Support Groups can be enormously beneficial, for obvious reasons. *Counseling* can provide stimulus and direction for those who falter.

Diet and Nutrition tells that eating well and sensibly is not only enjoyable but important, as is *Exercising* properly - another source of *Goals*, the setting of which is discussed early in the book. *Driving* is covered, too.

Additional very important strategies for improved well-being are described in *Special and Enjoyable Diversion,* as well as *Alternative and Complimentary Therapies*.

5 - POSITIVE GUIDANCE *THAT REALLY WORKS!*

In this chapter there are not only valuable suggestions but much helpful information distilled from research, plus very significant new, practical and *entirely original* methods I have discovered through constant experimenting that cannot be found elsewhere. They will be helpful to you when taking that difficult first step even when your feet want to "freeze", and will guide you in the simple techniques used to overcome hand tremor.

Additional scores of ideas conducive to cheerful living and common-sense goals are provided in later chapters, in which you surely will find several important to and compatible with your chosen direction into the future.

TAKING THE FIRST STEP

There are big problems starting the first step when it is associated with stress or urgency ("*Uh, uh! Stop"*), moving toward a dead-end (a corner?) or when we are contemplating the traverse of narrow or confined spaces (*"No! You can't go through there.")* and the feet "freeze" and refuse to move.

That doesn't have to happen. I have learned how to navigate such treacherous terrain, and am detailing in the following paragraphs a number of methods that can and will start your feet walking.

On the following pages are several useful discoveries that <u>*truly, really and honestly do work*</u>. But first, this CAUTION! <u>*Do not to try to take a step when leaning forward because weight will be on both feet*</u> and they cannot move. The same must be said for attempting to step sideways with a weighted foot, because the only possible result is a fall to that side.

If your feet are "frozen" when you are standing close to a sturdy object you can use for support (kitchen counter, table, back of chair, etc.), smile, because you can make them walk by doing the following:

Standing ERECT with head up and feet pointing ahead with one slightly to the back, place a hand on a sturdy object and relax for a moment. When ready, gently "push away" with the hand and you're off!

Sticky-tape short reminders (in color?) where you will be sure to see them.

When standing <u>with no solid support within reach</u> to use for "pushing off" with a hand as explained above, you nevertheless will be able to start walking by:

Pointing your feet where you want to go with one slightly in back, STAND LOOSELY ERECT a few seconds until you feel relaxed, then push ahead with the ball of your back foot while WILLING that foot to step ahead. Do the

same with the other foot, and begin stepping ahead.

It's surprising how strong "force of mind" is.

Here is another technique that works absolutely every time to release foot-freeze (I believe because it makes me stand up straight):

With feet pointing ahead and one slightly to the back, stand loosely erect with head up and bring thumbs together pointing down inside your beltline and relax a few seconds. When you feel comfortable, sweep your thumbs around to meet at the back and begin walking (With each step push ahead with the ball of the back foot to make it easier to take longer steps and walk more erect and smoothly.

For some reason that thumb-sweeping motion releases foot freeze instantly and is effective for me even if I just circle my hands around to the back outside my clothing, or with just one hand if the other is carrying something.

Important! When my legs are unwilling to move I just stand loosely and quietly ERECT a few seconds letting mind and body unwind until they are 'at ease'. Then I use one of the methods shown here and I can walk okay. Try it.

Still another method that works for me; Wad up a sheet of paper of some kind, toss it ahead of you and step toward it, repeating this routine by kicking the "target" ahead (with your cane, as an example) and stepping toward it. Sound strange? It works for me and may be helpful to others.

I have better success walking if my first step is a long stride rather than a short one. It just feels better and easier because my legs seem looser. Keep your feet fairly far apart, laterally (side-to-side), while walking to counter imbalance and a fall to the side.

When entering a doorway with a formidable floor joint of carpet-to-linoleum (door into bathroom) I have been stalled occasionally, even when applying the methods listed here, but now have found it helpful to cross *at an angle*.

Another technique that works well when I am stalled at a doorway is to reach as far up the door jamb as possible with one or both hands, and grip while pulling ahead gently. This makes us stand up straight. But, if the feet still are reluctant to get going it may help to "high-step" the first steps <u>by bringing knees upward</u>.

When you do well, smile and <u>reward yourself</u> with a well-earned and meaningful compliment.

I can truthfully report improvement in my walking following my neurologist's instruction to take one tablet of *Mirapex* before breakfast, one tablet mid-day and *one-half* tablet before or after dinner, in addition to one *Sinemet CR* both morning and evening). Also, now that I have added two teaspoons of *oral* Glutathione (obtained from Wellness Health – see Chapter 13) in fruit juice first thing in the morning, my walking has become better and the first step easier.

This may help: Walk with initial foot-pressure thrusting forward with the ball of your foot (that's across the front of your foot where the toes are), rather than starting off by hitting on the heel and rolling the foot forward, or walking flat-footed. You will be more erect, and forward movement really can be more fluid and easier to maintain.

Depending upon your condition, you may find walking *stiff-legged* will help you get going.

Sometimes, a rapid backward and/or upward movement of an arm will help you step out of a "freeze", similar to the "thumbs hooked inside the beltline and swept around to the back".

A cane used to propel (gently) from the back helps at any time. Always walk as erect as you can (taking deep breaths will make you stand straighter), and take long strides. Smile.

Even if you use a walker (which wants you to lean forward), won't you feel better about yourself when you try to walk as erect as you can? When you do, with your mind fixed on straightening up the body, your walk may very well improve – enabling you to get to the coffeepot quicker, even while you're sneakily reaching into the cookie jar. Try to hide your guilty smile.

Avoid *pivoting on a heel* when turning, particularly if you can't hang onto something stable. The result can be nasty. I say this because my balance is now compromised to the point I have to be very careful when on my feet, especially if I am working on a turn without support. So, I turn in place veeeery carefully, and slooowwly with mind on the feet.

Turning in *confined* areas such as in your home must be done often, and can be very frustrating. When unable to reach a support when you need to change direction, one method for turning when one's balance is not dependable is to stand erect with feet spaced comfortably apart while slowly and carefully using the *outside* foot to progressively step ahead in stages, while compensating with the *inside* foot by adjusting it backward to accommodate every change of direction made by the outside foot (like rotating in place?).

To illustrate, when turning clockwise, step ahead with the outside (left) foot and point it as much as is comfortable in the direction to be taken next. When your weight goes onto that foot, you will be facing in the direction toward which that foot is pointing and your inside foot can be brought backward to adjust (and increase the turn-angle if your balance permits).

It is sensible to *pre-place your feet* in your proposed direction of travel *before* arising from a sitting position (turn your body on the chair before pushing yourself up onto your feet). Now, when you are erect you'll be facing in the right direction, or close to it.

To make a "progressive walking turn" (what we are really doing here is *walking around a curved route*) without support from a fixed object, when you are on your feet and not yet facing your destination merely take the first step ahead and begin turning by using progressive "cross-angle-foot-placement" as you move ahead until facing your destination, having placed your weight onto that outer "cross-foot" to turn you in the new direction.

When you reach the end of a straight walk and you want to change direction, try turning by placing the "outside" foot, on which you will turn, at an angle well ahead and directly across your previous line of travel and pushing off with that foot in your new direction. If this doesn't work for you, try rocking *slowly* sideways as you turn, standing erect (not leaning forward) with feet well separated. Then push ahead with your outside (back) foot as given in previous paragraphs. Never cross one leg over the other when turning because you'll lose your balance.

It's very important *that we do not lean forward* when attempting to take the first step, because (from a purely mechanical standpoint) both feet almost surely will have weight on them. *If we attempt to step ahead, or especially aside, on a weighted foot, nothing good will happen and we may fall because that foot cannot move*.

Have you heard this before? It's worth repeating! When you arrive at any point at which you must change direction, such as into a hall from a room, thrust your outside foot well ahead into the new area, pointing it directly across your old line of travel, in the new direction of travel. This just might move you right through a doorway (etc.), and you now will be aimed in the right direction.

There are times you will become highly agonized and angry when your feet just won't do what you want, all of which is normal and expected from time to time. When you find yourself in that state of mind, just realize you're leaning forward rather than standing erect, or are not concentrating on what you must do at the time. What are you doing wrong? Relax to get your head on straight, then start again and do it right this time. Because you can!

You have noticed my suggestions that we smile often. This definitely will make us relax better and free the feet, while our company is responding with their own happy faces. It works!

Sometimes, when your feet feel frozen or glued to the floor, a lift of the toes may eliminate muscle spasms and the fear of falling, and you will be free to walk again.

Another helpful idea is to place a stick (yardstick?) on the floor ahead of you, to step across. Or, merely place pieces of masking tape on the floor for you *consciously* to step across. If your mind is focusing on something extraneous such as the stick or tape, perhaps your feet will move easier. Some suggestions call for walking along a line-ahead, rather than across your path.

Try *imagining* a line across the floor, and step across it (this way, you will be able to sit down easier, because you won't have a yardstick in your back pocket).

In kitchens we'll be doing much turning from our work to the fridge, stove, sink, etc., with the frequency of our movements tending to keep one's mind on our work and forgetting the feet. We must be careful, for this is a prime place to lose balance and fall. (My dented garbage can knows all about this stuff).

Repeating: Before turning your body toward the next destination, no matter how close, first support yourself with a hand on a counter or any other substantial thing, then ALWAYS turn your feet in the direction of travel, bring them fairly close together with one slightly ahead of the other, stand erect looking ahead (not down) facing your objective, then step out carefully pushing with the toes of the back foot while <u>pushing ahead</u> with a hand on that solid object in your direction of travel. This may be repetitious to the point of being tedious, but forgive me, for it works well.

Conversely, if the feet freeze when you are about to enter a doorway, it helps to reach ahead and grab the doorjamb. Then standing erect and using the directions given earlier, gently pull yourself forward and push ahead with your *back* foot to free that difficult first step. Push off against the jamb to continue moving after passing through the doorway.

Avoid wearing shoes or footwear with rubber or crepe soles, because, as intended, they tend to stick to the floor.

Avoid "side-stepping" to move laterally, because the outside foot you are trying to move may have weight on it and absolutely will not move. Instead, for example in the kitchen next to a counter, turn your feet in the direction of travel while supporting yourself with a hand on the counter and gently shove yourself ahead with that hand. *I know I've said all this before, but it really initiates forward movement easily* - furthermore, you'll look good to your admiring audience rather than stumbling and jamming your head into the fridge or cookie jar.

WALKING FOR EXERCISE

When distance-walking for exercise, there usually are few turns so one can walk purposefully. When changing direction and turning, if you don't feel comfortable with placing your outside foot well ahead directly across you line of travel and pushing off with it in the new direction, then pause and turn carefully with feet well apart (a cane, or lamp post for support will help here) and initiate your first step as described previously. Or, (repeating!) just place one foot ahead, cross-wise, and push away on it to get going in the new direction as described very carefully before, because it really works.

When you get going, stride with the longest steps you can, pushing off each step with the toes of the back foot, which translates into keeping your body more erect (try to overcome a stooping posture) looking up and ahead. Swing your arms freely while walking, to help maintain balance and lessen fatigue.

And, when walking, here's good advice: *Keep a pleasant expression! Smile.* It'll take your mind off your legs, which will permit your feet to move more freely. Other pedestrians will admire you and smile. Give them a nod and an appreciative grin. Passing motorists will honk in admiration and wave. Return the wave. Smile and wave at anyone who looks nice.

If doing so does not interrupt balance while distance walking, you may wish to hold and swing light dumbbells for additional exercise. Remember to take long steps, rather than shorties. Your legs will be happier that way, and it is pleasing to see how fast the trees move by with the little birdies chirping and singing all around. How your eyes will shine! Hallelujah! It's great to be alive!

You may find it helpful to have the support of a cane with a broad rubber tip while walking. This may take a bit of practice before your timing feels entirely comfortable, but you soon will graduate to the dignified appearance of a Johnny Walker Boulevardier. You'll look fine swinging your "walking stick". And, it is entirely affordable and portable. But you knew that.

WALKERS AND WHEELCHAIRS

By definition, walkers (I discuss the four-wheelers here) must be easy to push and turn, so alert care must be taken when we use them, because if not carefully controlled a walker can scoot away from us with embarrassing or even painful results. They have two large wheels that pivot with any change of direction with rotary (360-degree) casters, all fitted with ball or roller bearings that respond to the slightest pressure.

Thankfully, walkers have effective and easily-applied brakes that are operated simply by squeezing the brake lever on the handle. We must keep it in our grasp at all times when using our walkers. Even the teen-age show-off must grip the brake handle or risk doing cartwheels.

Walkers not only are user-friendly and very helpful, but for those of us who cannot turn safely without support are necessary *safety devices* in places in which we must turn often such as in the home, or in restaurants and other crowded areas. But they make us lean forward, a feature your neurologist and physical therapist may not favor because they want us walking as erect as possible, which our walker will not permit. Ask him, her or them. Whatever the case, I believe we always should endeavor to walk as erect as we can when using a walker.

A four-legged cane can be a useful device too, because it provides more support than a single-tipped cane, plus it can be stood upright next to you, within easy reach.

Don't overlook having your doctor <u>write a prescription</u> for a wheelchair, walker, cane <u>or any other</u> <u>assistive device</u>. <u>It will SAVE YOU MONEY</u> because your health insurance provider will pick up most or all of the tab.

If you served in the military, it may be a productive idea to check with the Veterans' Administration about providing some of your medical needs, <u>including medications at low cost</u>. The VA has been very helpful to me, and even provided the very finest hearing aids (both ears) at no cost to me.

HAND TREMOR

Hand tremor occurs when your arm is in its normal or usual position, with the twitching usually originating at the elbow and running down the forearm into your hand. When you twist (rotate) your hand into an *unusual* position, as discussed below, the wobbling *will stop.* Apparently, when certain muscles in your forearm are "torqued" into an unusual tension relationship, hand tremor will not be induced.

Each of the following suggestions should stop tremor while being maintained.

To relieve hand tremor in any position, spread and keep your hand wide open, then relax it and rotate the hand outward.

TO STOP HAND TREMOR, WHEN SEATED

To stop your hand wiggling, press your wrist or forearm against your thigh

Extend your arm forward, clench something in your fist (see ideas below), *rotate* your hand outward (inward may be just as effective) and hold it there.

Or extend and rotate it palm-up and hook your thumb under something solid (table next to your chair?) to prevent your hand from returning to its normal position. If there isn't anything close enough to use for this, put a heavy TV table or something similar next to your chair and use that.

Or, if you like far-out stuff and want to fabricate something that will keep your hand turned palm-up without any effort by you, cut the thumb off a large glove and with it stuffed full of paper or cloth wrap its end with several layers of lead strip (or attach something heavy to the tip). When it is slipped over the thumb of the offending hand, the weight must be heavy enough to pull your thumb down and keep that hand rotated palm-up on the arm of your chair.

Or extend your arm straight down over the side of the chair and rotate your hand outward and hook the thumb into or under something to prevent your hand from returning to its usual, normal position.

Or, thrust the offending hand palm-down under your thigh, where your weight will keep it from moving.

Get a spring-loaded hand exerciser, a tennis ball or a firm compressible ball that fits your hand, and keep it handy for steadily squeezing or alternately squeezing and releasing to relieve tremor. (Wonderful how your hand and forearm will strengthen).

If all else fails, stare at your hand and command it to stop. Sometimes this works.

STOP HAND TREMOR, WHEN STANDING

Put your arm around someone you love, smile and squeeze! Hard! Nuzzle a little. Do this often!

If your hand wiggles while you're standing, press your wrist against your thigh. If the tremor starts again, rotate your hand and press it against your thigh.

If you can reach something solid such as the back of a chair or a counter, grip it. Your hand cannot wiggle. Or grip something in your fist and hold it.

TO STOP HAND TREMOR, <u>WHILE WALKING</u>

While distance-walking for exercise and hand tremor is bothersome, although your arms are swinging, keep your hand in *anything other than its normal position,* such as rotating it outward. Or give it something else to keep its attention: Grip something in your fist (your thumb?), perhaps merely squeezing a leaf between thumb and forefinger, whatever you find effective at the time (a finger thrust through a dangling key-ring works well for me) and twist your hand clockwise and hold it (or counter-clockwise).

Your mind will be occupied with what's going on with the offending hand, which will free your legs to stride ahead very nicely. All who notice will applaud and loudly express their enthusiastic admiration until the cops arrive to investigate the disturbance - but you'll be long gone by then.

TO STOP HAND TREMOR, <u>WHILE LYING DOWN</u>

If you're trying to get to sleep, and tremor won't let you, *(This is very effective for me!)* lie on the same side as your wiggly hand, and thrust it between your drawn-up thighs (better yet, under a small pillow between your knees) where it will be held securely while you get to sleep. Palm-down is an unusual position and should do the job, but if not, turn it palm-up and spread wide. Whenever the fidgety mitt is not in its normal or usual position it will get so confused it will stop its tremor and we can drop off into the land of ZZZZ. There's no hand tremor while we're asleep!

When turning over, do the same on that side. If you are moved by a need for variety, consider sticking your offensive hand palm-up under your pillow, where it will be handy for scratching if something itches.

If you're lying on your back, your hand normally will be palm-down across your chest or resting next to you. Try stuffing it palm-up under your bottom or thigh.

If you're sleeping on your tummy, you can turn the offending hand into its unusual position, under your thigh or pillow where it will be held by your body weight.

LEG TREMOR

I do not have leg tremor, so cannot provide experienced ideas, but it makes sense to apply the facts learned about hand tremor: If the limb is turned or rotated into a posture that is *not usual or normal*, the tremor should stop. So, if I were seated or in bed and affected by leg tremor, I would rotate the foot involved and secure it comfortably under or back of something to hold it. This should work for legs as well as it does for hands. A thought: When walking, leg tremor should not be present, but I assuredly would not drive a car if either foot wobbled, because it may not perform when and as required.

SWALLOWING

I used to have swallowing problems, but was helped by the following information to the extent swallowing no longer is of much concern. Chewing and swallowing problems (there are specialists in this field) often can be met by practical recommendations which include taking small bites and eating slowly, swallowing only well-chewed food often to empty the mouth, and sipping a liquid (*through a straw while leaning forward slightly!*) before taking the next bite. I've learned it is necessary to have a cup or glass of water with a straw in it within easy reach when I need a sip or two to clear away food particles that sometimes get stuck in my throat and cause choking. Swallowing instruction can be provided by a Speech Therapist, or down-loaded from the internet.

If swallowing is a problem, perhaps you should use a blender to reduce hard-to-chew food into an easy-to-swallow consistency, while the flavor is retained.

As a precautionary measure, your caregiver (or family members) should be versed in the application of the *Heimlich Maneuver*, an emergency technique for preventing suffocation by dislodging an obstruction in the throat or windpipe, such as when a victim's airway or throat becomes blocked by a piece of food. It can be used safely on both adults and children, although most experts do not recommend it for infants less than one year old. *It also can be self-administered.* The Heimlich Maneuver is detailed in Chapter Nine.

Here's another very helpful suggestion that proved most helpful for me: If you have difficulty swallowing liquid, use a straw!!!! Hot/Cold flexible straws that bend close to one end are inexpensive and easy to find. Sip while leaning forward with chin down, to facilitate the liquid's sliding down the right pipe.

Another helpful suggestion: If you have trouble swallowing pills or capsules, pop a small amount of yogurt (or some other semi-liquid slippery stuff such as a mouthful of chewed-up food - bananas are super - ready to swallow) into your mouth, then put the pill or capsule in there with it and swish it around everything and lean forward with chin down, to swallow. This will "lubricate" the pill or capsule and make it much easier to swallow. Extra caution should be taken if you plan to swallow an unusually large capsule or pill, and you should ask your caregiver to be present in the event you choke.

If you chew pills, be sure you are not doing so to any CR (Controlled Release) or similar pills, because it destroys their time-release feature.

You may wish to quiz your doctor about this, for some pills don't work properly if cut or chewed (SineMet CR, for example).

Additionally, I have discovered a flavored drink eases pill-swallowing when sipped with a straw.

BREATHING

I have breathing difficulty typical of Parkinson's and other MDs, which often becomes labored, especially after awakening at night. But, GOOD NEWS! I have found a solid solution to the labored breathing problem that had affected me day and night. I discovered *"ClearLungs, Red Label"* hiding in the vitamin catalog and ordered a couple of 60-capsule containers. Immediately upon taking the first few capsules, my breathing was restored to about 60-70 percent *of normal.* So of course I am taking *ClearLungs (Red Label)* regularly now *(at first* two capsules three times daily with meals for 2 – 3 weeks to load up, now only one in a.m. and one in p.m. to "maintain"). It is an Herbal Supplement ("*Chinese Formula For The Lungs*") from Ridgecrest Herbals, 1151 S. Redwood Road, Suite 106, Salt Lake City, UT 84104*)* (*www.ridgecrestherbals.com.)*

There are several suppliers of similar herbal supplements one can access via the internet, so you should compare products and prices to be sure you have the best choice when you buy. Some sell RidgeCrest products – at a huge discount (buy two, get five)

This may help you too: When I wake at night I mix and sip a small amount of Ovaltine in hot milk, after which my breathing usually eases enough to let me sleep again. For this purpose my lovely care-giving bride of many years got me a little round hot plate that heats my milk on my bedside table while I sleep.

However, here is a solid suggestion based upon experience with my mug of HOT coffee in the morning: If you are seated and breathing is not easy, drink a hot beverage to considerably ease the throat and make breathing less constricted, then lean back a bit (a reclining chair is super here) and notice how good your breathing has become.

We know people with asthmatic attacks are relieved by breathing in a hot vapor (some call it "steam") laced with a medication. I don't know if a nasal inhaler will help, because I have not tried one. But ask your doc.

SPEECH

If we are having difficulty speaking *distinctly*, it's at least partly due to inattention to the basic modes involved. To minimize this condition (my speech therapist advises) we should exercise our talking apparatus *at least once a day* for five minutes, by talking aloud (read from a book) with all speaking motions greatly-exaggerated (mouth widening, jaw and tongue motions, etc.). For exercising voice power, shout into a pillow.

When speaking to another person, face your listener directly, emphasizing key words and using short sentences. If all this is done regularly, your speech will improve simply because the exercises will have become automatic features of your speaking.

SLEEPING WELL

PD and other medications often induce insomnia, the first symptom of which is difficulty getting to sleep. I have found a sensational way to overcome it merely by taking my evening PD pill (Sinemet CR) *just before bedtime.* I used to have insomnia almost every night, taking up to an hour or more to get to sleep and often getting only three or fours of sleep, total. Then I decided to take my dinnertime Sinemet CR before hitting the hay because I deduced my morning Sinemet CR pill must be the cause for my becoming very sleepy during breakfast. I now am asleep quickly and enjoy several hours of good sleep.

HANDWRITING

Usually goes haywire for ParkinPeople and those with similar Movement Disorders, and our hand will want to scribble more and more rapidly, with the writing line becoming progressively smaller. Don't let it. Our handwriting can be improved considerably merely by concentrating on writing slowly, *with the other hand steadying and stabilizing the writing hand.*

If your script still is poor and difficult to read, PRINT, slowly, using one hand to support and steady the writing hand. My handwriting has just about disappeared, so I am teaching my left hand to write. It's a gas!

GENERAL

When you're going to be sitting or lying down, before doing so be wise-and-ready by placing the telephone close at hand, so you won't have to struggle to your feet to reach the loud-mouth thing before the caller disconnects. Same with your cane, medications and glass of water, books, reading glasses, the TV remote control, and so on. If you're reading and the phone rings in the kitchen, too far to get to before it gives up on you and goes silent just before you grab it, don't blame me. Read the first part of this paragraph again.

When approaching a chair to sit down, place one foot close to the *far* side of the chair-front pointing straight ahead so you will be positioned normally before <u>leaning forward</u> to slowly and carefully deposit your wazoo onto that comfy seat. Sigh!

Before arising from a chair, draw heels back to the front edge of the chair with feet pointing in the direction of the proposed travel, then push/slide the body forward so it will be <u>right above</u> our feet when we come to the standing position. When arising we should first lean forward before strongly pushing upward and forward with our arms while thigh muscles propel us upright.

Our weight must be directly above the feet when arising from a chair or we will find ourselves seated again, suddenly. When seating yourself, remember to <u>lean forward</u> and support yourself with hands on the chair arms while delivering your bottom onto the chair, because you'll descend slowly and carefully that way (look before sitting to be sure nobody has placed your fine imported bonbons on the chair - nothing uglier than a squashed bonbon shrieking complaints in French).

When arising from a bed, there is much to be said for overcoming a sudden tendency toward light-headedness by moving slowly upright and sitting on the edge of the bed for several seconds before standing - then standing in place another few seconds to clear the head before starting to walk. This may have to be consciously practiced before it will become automatic, but it just may prevent dangerous falls.

It may be helpful to place blocks under the legs at the head of our bed, to elevate the head end and make it easier for us to sit up and swing our legs off the edge. Also, a knotted rope attached to the foot of the bed can help pull oneself up, as may a four legged cane standing straight up within easy reach to help us onto our feet.

For greater safety in the bathtub, place a chair or stool in the tub, with the legs cut off (if necessary) so the seat is level with tub sides. For easier access to the toilet, a raised seat may be helpful. These are commercially available, as are toilet armrests. Grab bars usually are imperative at both bath and toilet.

You may find use for other adaptive equipment: Vibrating seat and backrests that have heating elements and are light and portable; bed rails; wide-handled utensils; special kitchen assisting devices are numerous and super-helpful; sip cups; special clothing (with Velcro fastenings, pullovers, large buttons if not zippered, padded if and where needed); book holders; large-button phones, etc. Vendors' catalogs are ours for the asking via telephone or internet.

Caution: Remove all throw rugs and other dangerous floor items that can cause falls for the unwary, and repair or remove carpet/rug irregularly-raised sections. Door sills can be made less dangerous by installing on both sides gentle ramps carrying brightly colored, reflective stripping.

6 - SETTING GOALS

We humanoids by nature are goal-setting. This is good, for without goals how can we experience the satisfaction of *achievement*, which in itself will promote self-esteem? There are numerous opportunities for goals to be found within our range of objectives, such as in exercising, reading, walking (a mile?), writing an article or book, learning how to turn without imbalance, improving handwriting, painting or other artwork, sewing, and so many others you will think of if you try. We should start with easy-to-reach goals.

Sometimes, a goal can be overwhelming in its scope. Consider the Grand Canyon, and its having been formed by a thrifty Scot who lost a penny down a gopher hole.

Goals should be prioritized. Our most important goal should get the most attention and time spent, for it actually is an intellectual experience that affects our feeling of well-being. <u>Once gained, a goal becomes an achievement to be referenced with satisfaction and realization of added independence.</u>

Wouldn't itemizing goals be an important element in coping with our condition? Such a list would make necessary the prioritizing of the goals and careful planning to begin the process of working toward success.

Keeping the mind active is vital to our moving forward into a satisfactory future, for we must keep the mind working to maintain overall good health. An active and healthy mind helps to light the sparkle in the eyes and maintain good emotional balance in which optimism is foremost. We must practice our minds constantly by doing something that makes us think, like reading, writing, writing a book, playing games (this is a very good challenge for one's mind).

I'll bet you would be good at writing a book (for children? A family history?). First, outline the story, then gradually fill in the essentials. Now, actually write the full text chapter by chapter. After you're finished, go back over it several times to edit, fine-tune it and correct typos. Your local library will have a number of instructional books dealing with authoring.

A really good copy shop has all the equipment to not only produce all the text (including photo images, etc.), but can finish-bind the book in several ways. You will have to supply the "cover-art" for both front and back covers, and will be helped greatly by computer programs such as "WordArt", a wonderfully diverse assortment of elaborately colorful fonts produced by Microsoft in their "Office 2000" and other sources.

If you believe the book to have good commercial potential, you'll need an "ISBN" (International Standard Book Number - only one book in the entire world has your ISBN) or it won't be accepted by book stores or even libraries. The only USA provider (at a small charge) of ISBNs is R. R. Bowker (877-310-7333). And you should have a "Library of Congress Book Number", or a "Lib. Of

Congress Pre-publication Book Number". You can get these online, for free at the Library of Congress website - following the prompts.

Bowker will provide a list of agencies that supply *barcodes* for books, when they send you your ISBN(s). You must have a barcode containing the ISBN and retail price on the lower edge of the back cover, if the book is to be sold in stores, including Amazon, etc. The least expensive source is Bar Code Graphics, Inc. (800-662-0701) whose website permits ordering a barcode online for only $10.00, and they will e-mail your printable barcode wherever you direct.

If you want to turn the entire enchilada over to a commercial firm specializing in book publishing, you may elect to turn it over to a "Print-On-Demand" (POD) company. These shops use computerized printing to produce one or a million copies. A very good one is "iUniverse" (1-402-323-7800), a subsidiary of Barnes and Noble, the huge bookstore chain. iUniverse does excellent work and even supplies cover art design.

If your goal is to have your book published by a fine main-line publishing house, I strongly suggest you contact Tate Publishing Co., 127 E. Trade Center Terrace, Mustang, OK 73064. (888-361-9473) (www.tatepublishing.com) Tate will spend from $14,000 to $21,000 of its own money on each book to handle every aspect of publishing, distribution, publicity, etc., but requires an up-front "author investment" of $3,985, which is refunded when your book reaches 5,000 sales, and the author receives a case of free books and a lifetime

60% off book purchases. They also are providing a top-of-the-line audio book version of your work with no additional charge to the author. Tate selects only 4% of the 10,000 or more books annually received for consideration, and has been named a "Publisher of the Year".

Now that you have done the book-authoring thing, how about considering playing brainy games such as Bridge, or Cribbage - an easy game to learn and it's fast and fun (a cribbage board and a deck of regular playing cards is all it takes - very inexpensive and a great gift idea). Or Solitaire, for those who have no company at the time. And, good people, don't overlook learning how to use a computer, for it can bring countless hours of fun and diversion.

There are dozens and dozens of games that can be played on your computer. For example, "Hoyle Card Games" is a program with 16 games - all those you enjoy. It and other such game programs can be bought at any of several chain stores - or, on the cheap at "eBay" (the online auction website). There's another idea for a super gift for a MD person.

You might consider actually putting down on paper the music you have composed by just humming to yourself. It would help to have a piano, but if you live in an apartment, your next-door neighbor may object to your tinkling. If so, a keyboard would work there, however, because they are electronic with adjustable volume. And, they come with instructions.

Your local library surely has books on how to write music, graphically. Or, the music store has them for sale, along with printed blanks for composition. Try your local college or university music department for assistance. If you are gifted and have original music in mind, you should be aware this is a proprietary item, and you shouldn't even hum it within the hearing of others. Keep it to yourself until you have copyrighted your music immediately upon its graphic scoring. Even a short and light tune can be a hit!

Once you have composed a sonata, why not apply for a patent on that device you have had in mind for so long? You do not have to hire a patent attorney. I know all about this, as an inventor who has published a book on do-it-yourself patenting without an attorney.

Why not auction off some items of value you no longer need, on e-Bay or other online services (search the internet for "Auctions"). Go on-line and search for "e-Bay", and that site will guide your listings. If you are adept at this, you may find some modest employment in listing and selling un-needed but utilitarian items for friends who can't (no computer?) or will not be bothered with it, and taking a fair commission. If you do get into this, you'll find it engrossing and challenging.

Now may be the right time to finally get all those photo albums in order. This may take many days or weeks to accomplish, but somebody has to do it.

Get busy with pencil and paper and list everything you consider to be *delightful!* Keep at it and you may just discover diversions not already thought of, that you can (and will) use that truly will add enjoyment to your everyday life. What a fun and light-hearted way to spend some time, maybe with input from others.

Pull a cute surprise on someone you love, and you'll all laugh.

Perhaps you will (finally) learn that foreign language - Spanish? French? You can do this day-by-day via the internet, or by Teaching CDs (library has these) that are readily available at stores that sell computer program CDs. If not a foreign language, why not learn how to assist others with their tax returns? Or raise colorful fish for sale in your aquarium?

Planning ahead, doing artwork (art can be a wonderful goal), singing (church choir?), gardening and a myriad of other pursuits can be goals. Perhaps you would do well in volunteer work (can be done from your own home, too). Why not organize a group to make up and donate boxes of helpful things for shut-ins (contact churches, city and county agencies for information). Have you given thought to your becoming proficient in photography?

But on the other hand, watching TV programs doesn't require much if any mental gymnastics and the ads are - ugh! But, we do need to relax sometimes. Your TV cable company may offer extra channels that bring you a great variety of music, movies, sports, etc., or one can get set up with a "satellite dish" that is oriented to pick up TV signals from a satellite and will bring you a hundred or more additional channels beyond those provided by basic cable or other services.

Isn't it true that that people with high self-esteem and an optimistic attitude already will have developed a healthy determination to cope with a MD and sustain energy, activities and relationships that give life meaning and positive direction?

WHAT CAN YOU DO BEST?

DO IT!

7 - SPECIAL AND ENJOYABLE DIVERSIONS

PETS, PLANTS, BIRDS AND GUPPIES

There is so very much to be said for owning a pet!

Especially a canine-type pet! A puppy cannot be equaled for exuding love and affection. Is there anything to equal the laughter and joy in the wagging tail of a fluffy puppy when he looks at you with those adoring eyes and bounces up to you for some love? That will bring a big smile to anyone's face. [My wife works at a cosmetics counter in a large department store that caters to the up-scale trade, and once waited on a be-jeweled lady cuddling a pampered miniature poodle with its own be-jeweled collar. She called it *"Woo-woo"*].

A dog gives his master its absolute and unquestioned loyalty and devotion. All he wants to do is please his owner and will unhesitatingly give his life to protect his "daddy" or his "mommy". A dog is wonderful company, for it always will listen attentively when spoken to (while cocking the head from side to side), and doesn't "talk back".

Cats make comfortable company, too, and don't bark and keep you awake at night, because they probably are quietly hunting mice. They too, enjoy a scratch, especially on the back. A cat with a fancy collar is a cat that owns its owner.

You might wish to make your selection at the local animal shelter and save the life of an animal you will come to love, if you can resist the temptation to take *all* those pleading doggies and kitties.

> Did you know there are Service Dogs available for MD patients? Try *Independence Dogs for the Mobility Impaired* - (610) 358-2723. 146 State Line Road, Chadds Ford, PA 19317 http://www.independencedogs.org

Other pets can be important to our inner health, too, such as birds, of which there are several varieties for our enjoyment. A canary's song will bring delight to an entire household. But the parrot you buy from a pet store may be second-hand and taught to say naughty things and always talks back, sometimes with colored language you don't really need when your very-proper bridge-and-tea ladies are present.

There is a story about a young bachelor who acquired a parrot from the local pet store just before Thanksgiving. As soon as he got it home and had set the bird-cage in the living room of his small apartment he heard cussing he couldn't believe was coming out of a bird. Soon he'd heard enough and stuffed the loud-mouth feathered thing into the fridge to cool off. The parrot squawked and shrieked for a few seconds, then there was complete silence. When he had heard nothing from his expensive parrot after several minutes, the young man thought it might be dying and opened the fridge door. There sat the huddled bird at the front of the middle shelf, looking up at his new master as it murmured: *"If you'll take me out of this frigid hell-hole, I promise never, never to cuss again. But I have a question. What did that poor turkey do?"*

There are quite a few choices when considering a pet. Why not visit a pet store and see all the animals, and the birdies, and so many other companions? Don't overlook an aquarium with pretty guppies, for it can bring endless fascination to the viewer. And fishies don't talk back, either. If they do you'd be well advised to back away, because it's the wrong kind of fish and you're in trouble!

All people enjoy and marvel at the beauty of flowers, especially those planted and nourished into blossom by you, outdoors and indoors. Indoor flowers take little space and are easily maintained. A home with flowering plants tells of comfort and happiness. Also, don't forget the non-flowering plants such as *ficus* and others that can fill a corner with Nature's beauty.

Happy companions like these little guys will brighten our days.

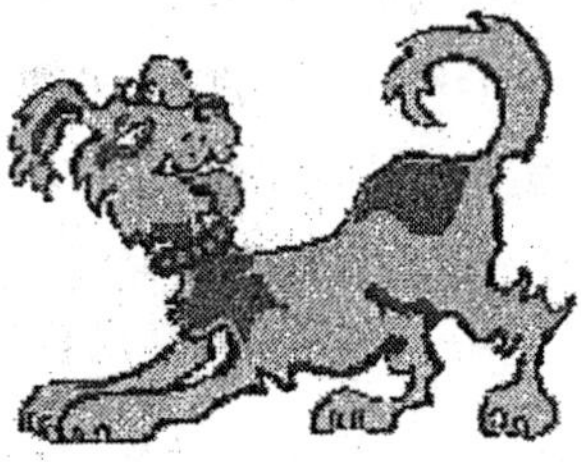

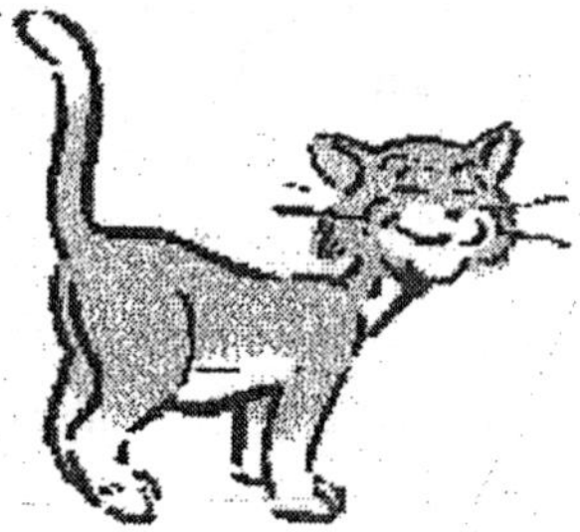

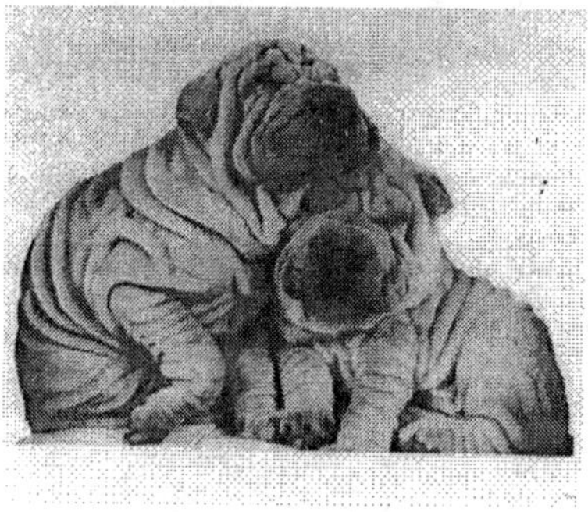

puppy-love!

8 - SUPPORT GROUPS

Attendance at MD support group gatherings can really be enjoyable and helpful through interaction with others who are similarly affected. The discussions can be between just two people, several or the entire assembly, and are entirely frank, open and in good spirit. Ask your physician about this. He/she should be the first to suggest, no, *insist,* that you contact your local support group and become involved. It's excellent therapy!

You usually can locate this local group by its listing in the yellow pages, *or by information provided by your physician.* Or, if you have a PC (personal computer) you can go on-line to search for and pull up one of the *Parkinson's, Dystrophy, Huntington's, Stroke, etc. Support Groups* in your city or county. Adding your city, county or state will narrow the search and you'll have the information quicker. The internet is absolutely fabulous, and it will come up with what you want even if your search-subject is vague.

If you don't own a computer or have no access to a friend's or relative's, try your local library. Most libraries have several PCs with internet access, for use by members at no cost.

Sometimes, the County will have the upper hand and functions as "Supervisor", etc., with the local support groups listed in its website.

Whatever the situation, the name and phone number of the person heading the local support group will be shown, for easy access. All MD people are welcomed with open arms, and usually at no cost or a very low fee to cover postage and copying of meeting notices.

The members of the support group, you will find, are utterly friendly and you'll make friends quickly and painlessly among them for this spirit is very contagious! Interchange of information is exceptional and beneficial. Meetings are held in any of several places such as homes, church meeting rooms, restaurants, etc.

Your support group almost surely will sponsor enjoyable times such as pot-luck meals, maybe with fun movies, too. And, often, guest speakers will be brought in, who will bring news of new treatments and other pertinent subjects. And, there are homemade cookies, cakes and soft drinks!

If there is no support group near you, why not learn how many people with your illness live within a few miles, and organize a new group? Your physician(s) may help with names and addresses after they obtain the consent of their patients.

For our kind of people, both updated information and social interactions are key factors in maintaining a positive attitude. Though we may seek these through traditional means such as our doctors, families and friends, you also may turn to the internet through which medium you may compare notes with other patients by subscribing to an Internet mailing list. Some of these deal with PD, for example, as only one of a number of MD and other neurological disorders, while others may focus on care-giving.

One such website is an open forum just for PD patients - "PARKINSN" - which is maintained at the University of Toronto, and through which you may pose questions or just let off some steam. You will see any kind of messages relating to exercises that can relieve discomfort, surgery success, stories, book reviews, poems, even some PD jokes. (One list member announced he is marrying his doctor and invited everyone on the list to his wedding). Now, that's a joyful bit!

To join "PARKINSN" send an e-mail to: *LISTSERV@LISTSERV.UTORONTO.CA,* saying in the body of your note: "subscribe PARKINSN (then your first name) (then your last name)"

If you search the internet, you can find several sites that provide "chat rooms" dedicated to a certain illnesses, where you can trade "online" questions, information, etc. And very possibly, make new friends.

9 - CAREGIVERS

If you are fortunate enough to have your spouse as your caregiver, count your blessings. If not, you may be favored by having the attendance of a relative or neighbor or friend. Otherwise, you can arrange for assignment of a caregiver through a local agency sponsored by your State.

The Personal Assistance Exchange for disabled assistance users and assistants is sponsored by the Independent Living Institute, website is: (*www.independentliving.org*) and assists in job opening searches, and in finding nannies, maids, sitters, etc., with thousands of USA names with resumes to match.

NATIONAL ASSOCIATION FOR HOME CARE is located at: 228 Seventh Street, SE, Washington, D.C. 20003. Phone: (202) 547-7424. NAHC is departmentalized:; Center for Health Care Law, Exhibiting, Hospice, Legislative, etc.

NATIONAL FAMILY CAREGIVERS ASSOCIATION is a large organization, and can be reached at: Suite 500, 10400 Connecticut Ave., Kensington, MD 20895-3944. Phone: 1- 800-896-3650. E-mail: *info@thefamilycaregiver.org*. They supply many services.

There are many caregiver websites that are immediately accessible by all of us (remember the library PCs if you have no computer). Some are professional while others are not.

Try the yellow pages in your phone book, or ask your physician for direction. Your friends in the local support group can provide a wealth of information on who and where to contact on this matter. If no luck here, go online and search *"Parkinson's Caregivers"*.

You'll come up with websites for the following and many others:

- Family Caregiver Alliance
- Christian Caregivers
- Caregivers-USA
- Empowering Caregivers
- Caregiver Media Group

There are many vendors' websites such as "*CaregiverProducts.com*" where you can order on-line the items you need, or to arrange for product catalogs to be mailed to you.

Now then, you should know of the possibility your non-professional caregiver such as your ever-loving spouse is eligible to receive substantial stipend for being your caregiver. This helpful income is available, for the most part, to people with low incomes. The criteria for eligibility will be stated at the outset, or the person manning the provider phone will discuss this issue with you.

If your support group cannot help you on this, start by contacting the Social Security Administration for initial information on all aspects of *caregiver financial assistance.* Then turn to your State for details on its participation in the caregiver's program. Some states have more than one funding program. Some programs will require a partial assumption of monetary benefits by the caregiver/patient, or may provide all funding.

Running down the information you need may take some time and try your patience, but if you need such monetary assistance or could use some help with costs, etc., don't delay, delay. Get on the ball and learn all about your and your caregiver's eligibility, plus the range of benefits available to you. You may be very pleasantly surprised.

Your caregiver should know how to do the Heimlich Maneuver. This life-saving procedure is applied to victims of choking (conscious or unconscious), asthma, or drowning.

For adults who are choking: From behind, wrap your arms around the victim's waist, make a fist and place it with thumb side against the victim's upper abdomen, below the ribcage and above the navel. Grasp your fist with other hand and press into upper abdomen with a quick upward thrust. Do not squeeze the ribcage, but confine the force of the thrust to your hands. Repeat until object is expelled.

If the victim is unconscious, or the rescuer cannot reach around the victim, place the victim on back. Facing the victim kneel astride his/her hips, with one of your hands on top of the other, place the heel of bottom hand on upper abdomen below rib cage and above the navel. Using body weight press into victim's upper abdomen with quick upward thrust. Repeat until object is expelled. If the victim has not recovered, proceed with CPR and call 911 for medical assistance. (Don't slap the victim's back – this could make matters worse).

For applying Heimlich to yourself, make a fist and place the thumb side of the fist against upper abdomen, below ribcage and above navel. Grasp your fist with the other hand and press into upper abdomen with a quick upward thrust. Repeat until the object in your throat is expelled. Your medical book must include the HM.

Don't overlook the possibility the patient may be eligible for *early or special* Social Security benefits (this is detailed in the following chapter). Check it out. Also, many medical expenses are tax-deductible, and may help to reduce taxes or effect larger tax refunds.

10 – MOVEMENT DISORDER RESOURCES

MEDICARE MODERNIZATION ACT (MMA)

The MMA (passed by Congress in 2004) established a privately administered prescription drug benefit that will become effective on January 1, 2006. It is called Medicare Part D Prescription Drug Coverage. The old plan ends on December 31, 2005. The Part D plan is quite complicated and will not be detailed here due to this complexity. To learn all about it, you may find it necessary to ask your pharmacist for printed matter describing it in detail, before making the decision to or not to enroll.

If you have internet access, go to: http://www.medicare.gov and follow the prompts for the information you need.

If you are eligible for both Medicare and Medicaid, you are a "dual eligible" person. And if you are a Dual Eligible with disabilities, you usually will receive Social Security and Medicare benefits, plus Supplemental Security Income and Medicaid benefits. Note: If you received a "CMS Medicare & You" handbook in the mail in October, 2005, you should know it contained a significant error affecting daily eligible beneficiaries. Get the corrected version before spending any time on it.

ORGANIZATIONS, ETC.

There are many organizations, foundations, government projects, etc., directed toward assistance for MD folks of all types, for which information is available online or via library sources or medical personnel. There are thousands of federal, state and local government agencies, non-profit organizations and commercial services. But, there are a number of key national and state agencies and organizations that can help people with disabilities negotiate their way through this maze of resources. One is described in the following data on RESNA:

A highly interesting, and possibly vitally important Federally-funded project is headquartered at: RESNA Technical Assistance Project *("RESNA" is the acronym for Rehabilitation Engineering and Assistive Technology Society of North America),* at 1700 No. Moore Street, Suite 1540, Arlington, VA 22209-1903. Phone is (703) 524-6686 and their direct E-mail is: *resnaTA@resna.org.*

RESNA's primary work is with people and companies designing and producing *highly technically-advanced* wheelchairs that make local transport possible for people with extensive handicaps, who otherwise would be unable to find a device that is responsive to their most minute direction through voice, finger touch, toe/foot touch, etc. If you need such assistive devices, you should contact the RESNA office in your own state.

The good news is this: All States, D.C., Northern Mariana Islands, Puerto Rico, the U S Virgin Islands and Samoa <u>are funded</u> under this Assistive Technology Act of 1998. The State offices are located in their capitol cities, and can be reached through the Federal Offices portion of our phone directories ("RESNA Technical Assistance Project").

The Alliance for Technology Access (ATA) is a large coalition of assistive technology programs throughout the USA. To learn if there is an ATA program near you, check the list of centers of ATA Centers on the Alliance's website. Or, your state may have a listing in the phone book, perhaps under "Assistive Technology; State Resources".

ABLEDATA maintains an online database of over 20,000 assistive technology products, and provides related information.

FOR CHILDREN

Focusing on children from birth to age 22, the National Information Center on Children and Youth with Disabilities (NICHCY) is a national clearing-house on information about disabilities and disability-related issued for families, educators and other professionals. NICHCY staff will walk you through the service maze and provide guidance and informational materials relating to early intervention, education, health care resources, legal rights, and many other concerns.

Additional resources: *Just For Parents (and Service Providers); State Resources.*

FEDERAL RESOURCE CENTER FOR WOMEN WITH DISABILITIES

This resource has been added to the National Women's Health Information Center, which functions as a single gateway to thousands of federal and private sector publications and organizations on women's health, through its website (http//www.4woman.gov) and toll-free information number (1-800-994WOMAN).

FINANCIAL ASSISTANCE

Social Security Disability Insurance (SSDI) is available to eligible workers with disabilities and their children or surviving spouses, who have Social Security coverage. The Social Security Disability Planner will guide you through this process.

Supplemental Security Income (SSI) is for people with little or no income and resources, regardless of Soc. Sec. Coverage or disability. Social Security's Supplemental Security Income pages will tell you more about this resource.

Medicare is a Federal health insurance program for people over 65 (Congress may change this upward) and people with disabilities of any age.

Medicaid is a Federal-State assistance program that pays medical bills of low-income people of all ages. The National Association of State Medicaid Directors provides a List of State Medicaid Web Sites.

Many of the resources listed elsewhere on these pages can provide financial assistance related to their areas. For example, some state Tech Act programs offer low-interest loans for assistive technology. Some vocational rehabilitation programs will pay for computer equipment, adaptive vans, and even personal assistants if they are necessary for your work. Your local independent living center may be aware of these and other funding resources in your own community.

HIGHER EDUCATION AND VOCATIONAL SERVICES

The HEATH RESOURCE CENTER is a national clearinghouse on postsecondary education for individuals with disabilities. HEATH serves as an information exchange about educational support services, policies, procedures, adaptations, and opportunities at American campuses, vocational-technical schools, and other postsecondary training entities.

Every state has a Department of Vocational Rehabilitation (VR) which helps adults with disabilities prepare for employment. The VR may provide medical, therapeutic, counseling, education, training, and other support services. The National Clearinghouse of Rehabilitation Training Materials provides a complete list of state VR agencies. Also, the State Rehabilitation Advisory Council for BVS of Pennsylvania lists state VR agencies on its website.

HOUSING

Affordable housing may be available through public housing, privately owned subsidized housing, or "Section 8" housing. Check your phone directory for your local public housing agency (PHA) or contact the U.S. Dept. of Housing and Urban

Development (HUD) 24-hour Housing Counseling Referral Line online or by calling 800-569-4287.

The U.S. Dept. of Housing and Urban Development also provides information about fair housing laws and other resources for people with disabilities.

INDEPENDENT LIVING

Independent Living Centers (ILCs) help individuals with disabilities live independently in the community through information and referral, skill training, advocacy, peer support, systems change, and other community-based programs. There are hundreds of ILCs throughout the country. To find one near you, contact the Independent Living Research Utilization Project (ILRU) and/or the National Council on Independent Living (NCIL).

LEGAL RIGHTS

Americans With Disabilities Act Disability and Business Technical Assistance Centers (DBTACs) provide information, referral, technical assistance, and training on the Americans With Disabilities Act (ADA) to businesses, state and local governments, and individuals. Call v/tty 800-949-4232 to be automatically routed to the DBTAC in your region.

Every state has a Protection and Advocacy (P&A) system which helps resolve problems and provide legal and advocacy counsel and litigation for eligible individual with disabilities. To find the

P&A in your state, contact the National Association of Protection and Advocacy Systems (NAPACS).

Each state has a Client Assistance Program (CAP) which helps individuals seeking or receiving vocational rehabilitation services. Contact NAPACS to locate the CAP in your area.

THE DRM WEBWATCHER

Useful for those with internet access, the DRM Webwatcher is a subject guide to the best disability resources on the Internet, and features hundreds of topics and disabilities with links to the best web sites. It will provide locations of organizations serving your own state and locality. You can learn all about this service by going to :*www.disabilityresources.org.*

"WE MOVE" is the name of an important organization that is dedicated to "Worldwide Education and Awareness for Movement Disorders" headquartered at 204 West 84th Street, New York, NY 10024. Their website is; www.wemove.org and e-mail: wemove@wemove.org. They assist those with Movement Disorders, and periodically prepare pertinent informative material concerning diagnosis and treatment of various MDs, as well as reporting on studies and their findings that they will send via e-mail to their subscribers. Be sure you are on their list.

There are several online sources of helpful information, among which is the Neurology Channel (search for it under that name), that is voluminous in its scope of the MD diseases. If you want information about a specific disease, search for it by name.

RESOURCES LIST FOR PARKINSON'S DISEASE

I went online and found a Resource List for ParkinPeople, that supply information on the illness, data on support groups, etc., and many provide literature that will be mailed upon request. Here are several:

My Parkinson's Info,
45 West 9000 South, Suite 2,
Sandy, UT 84070
Website: *www.myparkinsonsinfo.com*
Email: *mnilsen@myparkinsonsinfo.com*
This organization puts out a free monthly online newsletter that is packed with helpful info.

National Parkinson Foundation, Inc.
Bob Hope Parkinson Research Center, 1501 N. W. Ninth Ave. (Bob Hope Road), Miami, FL 33136-1494. (800) 327-4545.
Website is: *<http://www.parkinson.org>*.
Email:*mailbox@parkinson.org*
<mailto:mailbox@parkinson.org>.

Michael J. Fox Foundation For Parkinson's Research
Grand Central Station, P. O. Box 4777, New York, NY 10163. (800) 708-7644.
Website is: *<http://www.michaeljfox.org>*.

World Parkinson Disease Association
Via Zuretti, 35, 20125 Milano, Italy. (39) 02 66713111.
Website:*<http://www.wpda.org>*. Email: *info@wpda.org <mailto:info@wpda.org>*.

Parkinson's Resource Organization
74-090 El Paseo, Suite 102, Palm Desert, CA 92660-4135. (760) 773-5628 or toll free: (877) 775-4111. E-mail:*copsca@gte.net <mailto:copsca@gte.net>*.
Website: *<http://www.parkinsonresource.org>*.

The American Parkinson's Disease Association
1250 Hylan Blvd., Suite 4B, Staten Island, NY 10305-1946. (800) 223-3732 or (718) 981-8001.
Website: *<http://www.apdaparkinson.com>*
Email:*info@apdaparkinson.org <mailto:info@apdaparkinson.org>*.

Parkinson's Disease Foundation
William Black Medical Building, Columbia-Presbyterian Medical Center, 710 West 168th St., New York, NY 10032-9982. (800) 457-6676 or (212) 923-4700
Website: *<http://www.pdf.org/index.cm>*
Email: *info@pdf.org <mailto:info@pdf.org>*.

The Parkinson's Institute
1170 Morse Avenue, Sunnyvale, CA 94089-1605. (800) 786-2958 or (408) 734-2800.
Website: *<http://www.parkinsonsinstitute.org>*

National Institute of Neurological Disorders and Stroke
P.O. Box 5801, Bethesda, MD 20824
www.ninds.nih.gov <http://www.ninds.nih.gov>

Parkinson's Support Groups of America
11376 Cherry Hill Road, No. 204,
Beltsville, MD 20705 Phone: (301) 397-1545

United Parkinson Foundation
833 W. Washington Blvd., Chicago, IL 60607
(312) 733-1893
email:*upf_itf@msn.com <mailto:upf_itf@msn.com>*

DOCTORS' MEDICAL CENTER. FOUNDATION

There are many affiliates directly related to this foundation, that provide such valuable assistance as *Adult Day Health Care* (Nursing, Phys. Therapy, Speech Therapy, Psychosocial Services, Recreational and Social Activities, Support Groups, Healthy Meals and Snacks, Transportation, etc.) to those with needs deriving from Alzheimer's and related dementia.

There are numerous other MD resources that can be accessed by name of illness via the internet, that supply publications or online support (such as "chat rooms" mentioned earlier). Also of importance are resources similar to the listings for: *"National Parkinson Foundation Centers of Excellence"*, that are accessible by internet, and found in most of the states.

For Assistive Devices and such other helpful things such as special clothing, call those vendors listed in your yellow pages or go online to search.

You can find Doctor Referral services, probably in your yellow pages, and surely on the internet. The same applies to locating sources for assistance in Sleep Disorders, Incontinence and Depression.

Did you know you can even check on the records of "Bad Doctors"? Here is both phone number and website:
Questionable Doctors Listing,
(202) 588-1000.
Website:*<http://www.questionabledoctors.org>*

11 - EXERCISE

***Consistent* exercise is best, but *some* exercise is far better than none.**

Problems that respond well to keeping our physical selves in good condition through exercise are several and important:

Motor functions
Balance
Posture
Gait
Mobility
Maintain/increase activity level
Decrease rigidity and bradykinesia
(involuntary movements)
Facilitate movement and flexibility
Optimize gait

All the above plus other features you can think of will maximize independence, safety and function. Exercising will facilitate active movement, maximize fine motor coordination (eye-hand-body-legs) and improve endurance, plus, plus, plus *will improve your body image, self-esteem and psychological adjustment.*

Some folk will balk at flexing their muscles and exercising as much of their bodies as conditions permit, but they do so at their own risk! Others will enjoy bringing their physical beings into good condition, and will do whatever exercising their individual conditions permit, hopefully two or more times a week, if not at a gym then at home where it can be done daily.

> *However, before beginning a program or routine of exercising,* ***ask your doctor*** *for his/her approval, especially if you are taking a medication that changes your pulse rate, or if you have a pacemaker, or if you have atrial fillibration.*

HEALTH CLUBS (GYMS)

There are several beneficial "resistance" (using weights) exercises one can do at home, which will be described later. But if possible, I highly recommend working out in a gym ("health club", as some are called). Memberships usually are inexpensive. Not only do they have a multiplicity of machines and equipment, but most have one or more "trainers" who will start the beginner on appropriate moves, and who will instruct you on proper warm-up stretching exercises (they may suggest a few minutes on the rowing machine). Always do warm-ups first, and it's a good idea to do cool-downs, too, after your workouts.

An item of interest: I am 86 at this writing, and have been active in sports all my life until fairly recently, but have no joint problems (yet?). I suggest a good reason for this is my taking, for many years, a daily dose of Joint Maintenance preparations that contain a formulation of the Important-Three: Glucosamine Sulphate, MSM and Chondroitin Sulphate. (plus several other helpful elements). These preparations are touted not only to help provide joint lubrication but to re-build cartilage. And they are inexpensive!

I arbitrarily quit driving recently, because my Parkinson's medication seemed to make me light-headed at times, so I stopped before I did something bad. Because I am unable to drive myself to the gym nowadays and my lovely five-days-a-week-on-the-job-care-giver-bride cannot haul me there every other day, I do a full and entirely-satisfactory workout at home – see the following at-home workout menu.

I like the idea of going to a gym because everything we need is right there, and we can become friendly with others of our age and physical capability, who can be even more helpful than the trainers because they're personal and interested in our progress.

As ancient as I am, I have worked out in gyms for years, not only to "maintain" but to make me feel good. The people around me (just as many women as men) all are intent upon their personal workouts, and don't care who I am, what I'm doing or how I'm doing it.

So, if you are shy about getting started in a gym, know this: You can be sure nobody will even notice you unless you ask a question on *"how to"* or *"please spot for me while I use this equipment".* Then, the person to whom you have turned will stop his/her routine and give you every little bit of personal and friendly advice. Makes him/her feel useful, important and like a Good Samaritan.

When I ask a powerful young man for advice or assistance, he'll consider even an old guy like I am to be a mutually-involved buddy and will go the limit to help. (I get friendly with all the huge and powerful guys because if I get into a beef, I want them on *my* side).

A newcomer to a gym should not be self-conscious because nobody will do more than glance at you. They actually will *admire* older or infirm people just for being there and "doing it", and are not slow to compliment you. It happens.

If you are in poor physical shape and want to begin working out in a gym, but feel strange about the whole thing, I suggest you find a workout partner who is about your equal so you can share workouts and (importantly) encourage each other's attendance. It's really enjoyable when you have good company, with mutual congratulations for progress.

You don't have to lug around heavy "plates" while using the "free weights" like barbells, because many pieces of equipment are "cable" machines, which have stacks of small weights and use pins to select however many weights are desired, and have seats. Start with low weights and do plenty of repetitions using multiple leg and arm muscles, lower back, abdominal "crunches". You can set goals to make this really enjoyable by keeping a record of each workout so you can exult in positive progress. And you feel so much better. Now your eyes really are shining!

Don't overlook *cardio-vascular* and/or *aerobic* workouts! Ask your doctor before beginning such exercising, however, for you may be told to do water aerobics instead of the much more demanding alternative. Think about this carefully, since water aerobics are less demanding but beneficial, anyway. However, your doc almost surely will approve your using *cardio-vascular* equipment, even on a reduced scale to begin with.

All gyms have several, or many, machines for cardio exercise that address the entire body, even rowing machines. They are easy to use and important for maintenance of cardio-vascular health.

Your *aerobics* goal should be working up to 20 minutes or more of sustained moving, 3 times a week. (Perhaps your gym runs a regular aerobic class?). Begin by doing 3 - 5 minutes of *warm-up* - you can do this by marching in place or walking around the block. Finish your routine with a 3 to 5 minute *cool-down,* perhaps by continuing your activity at a lower pace or switching to a different activity.

Measures of rating how hard one is working are (1) The Target Heart Rate, which involves quite a bit of math, and (2) The Borg Rating Scale that increases exertion rating from "Very, very light" to "Very light", "Fairly light", "Somewhat hard", "Hard", "Very hard", "Very, very hard" to "Maximum Effort". Judge your own effort, but you surely won't be interested in going beyond "Somewhat Hard", will you?

EXERCISING AT HOME

To do strength exercises at home, you really don't need much equipment. Simple devices are available such as ankle and wrist strap-on weights with Velcro closures, hand-held dumbbells of many sizes and elastic resistance bands (cables). But wait – if you want to save a trip or two to locate and purchase these things, read on. Aha!

Actually, you can do several valuable moves using only sturdy one-gallon (or larger) plastic water bottles, filling them only with enough water to provide the resistance you want, to accomplish the several exercises below.

Do's and Don'ts for strengthening exercises:

Do work one muscle group at a time.

Do stop any exercise that causes pain.

Do perform the movements slowly.

Do concentrate on standing up straight while doing standing exercises.

Do breathe in while lifting, and breathe out when lowering weights.

Don't grip hand weights too tightly.

Don't do rapid or jerky movements.

Don't hold your breath. Breathe evenly throughout each exercise.

Do two or three "sets" (of several "repetitions" each) for all exercises.

Biceps - stand erect and lift the bottle by its handle in front of you up to your chest (if you have two bottles, then you can do both arms at the same time).

Shoulders - stand erect and lift the bottle along your side up into your armpit. You should be able to use considerably more weight on this one because you're using larger muscles that run from shoulder to neck.

Backs of arms - with one knee and hand on bench (bed will work), with arms fully extended and stiff, push bottle from floor backward, waist high.

Shoulders - same position as previous, but pick up weight from floor by pulling straight upward to chest.

Shoulders - holding bottle (or strap-on weight) next to hip and arm straight and stiff, lift weight outward up to shoulder level.

Lower back (if this hurts, don't go there) - bend over forward and with both hands gripping the bottle, lift bottle stiff-armed from floor using only lower back muscles.

Legs - Sit on something fairly high with weight attached to your ankle. With foot on floor slowly "kick" foot upward until fully extended and leg is horizontal.

Legs - Same as last or standing erect if possible, lift knee straight up with weight attached to foot, high as possible. Sure this smarts the lower abdomen, too, but just think how good it'll feel when you stop.

Legs (will this ever stop?) - With weight on floor, squat with feet about two feet apart, keeping back erect grab weight with both hands. Now, keeping back erect, push up with your thigh muscles until you are standing with the weight hanging from your hands, in front (Of course. If it comes up somewhere else, sir, you've got problems).

Given time, the last one will strengthen your thigh muscles, especially, so you'll be able to get up from a sitting position more easily. You really should do as many reps as possible, perhaps repeating the exercise two, three or more times with several reps each.

Legs (gotta do the legs because we need strong legs for walking and stuff) - Standing facing a wall with toes about a foot away from the wall (and supporting yourself with one hand gripping something like a door jamb, if necessary) do toe raises, all the way up. Must feel stress in your calves or you're not lifting your heels high enough. Do plenty of these, maybe two or three times (called "sets") of several "repetitions" each.

Legs (groan!) - We must do something about those slack and weak hamstrings (back of thighs), and you can exercise them by wrapping a strap/Velcro or other weight around the ankle and thrusting up and back from a crouched position. Don't try this with both legs at the same time, especially on your front lawn because you will stop traffic. (Maybe you could charge for admission).

Or, get a strong elastic cable loop and attach it to a baseboard if possible, or maybe around a chair-leg with your ever-loving darling sitting in it (to anchor it). Hook your heel (Achilles tendon) into the loop and pull it backward, away from its anchor until taut. Now, pull your foot backward as far as you can, then ease your foot forward again until the elastic cable loosens, then do it all over again and again and again. This will get your hamstrings right where they live, and they'll thank you forever for making them strong, even if you are wheezing at the time.

Legs! What? Again? Oh yes. But this one is easy. Lie on the floor on a small exercise mat, or on your bed. Lie first on one side, then the other while lifting your stiffened uppermost leg upward several times (you can attach an ankle weight, if you feel strong enough). This will strengthen the outer side of your thigh. Alternatively (to work the inside of your thigh) lying on one side then the other, lift the down leg up-down, up-down, up-down. Many times.

Legs. Again? You can't be serious! I'm not, and we're finished for the day. But tomorrow's another day, as they say.

An MD patient, no matter how severely affected, can do multiple exercises - even in a wheelchair. Example: Stiffen one leg at a time, straight out, then raise and lower it until you've had enough for that time. Stiff-arm raises to the side and to the front, then upwards close to the body, from floor to armpit (perhaps holding some kind of weight) can be beneficial. The armchair athlete can even do neck exercises, and can benefit the abs by merely sucking in the gut - repeatedly and strongly.

Everybody, those in wheelchairs, etc., and even those hardy folk who visit the gym every other day (really should rest a day or two after each resistance-training workout that uses the same muscles) will benefit by doing even a few stretching and abdominal drills immediately upon arising and especially before breakfast (the body has "fasted" ever since dinner the evening before, and lacking digested food will pull down fat for energy when stressed by exercise).

I like the following few drills that take only about 9-12 minutes, and do them absolutely every day when I get up (right after giving my scalp a heavy workout to save my hair). These alone will help keep you in good physical condition and feeling well, so please, please do the following 1 - 8 exercises *first thing* when you have eased yourself out of bed. If you are not in good physical shape, but start this simple regimen tomorrow morning and continue it for just three or four weeks, you will feel so much better you will never stop (because that would make you a quitter, and we can't have that).

1) Lying on your back across the bed (anyone can lie on a bed), do some stretching moves - pull knees up, one at a time, close to chest and hold with hands back of knee for half a minute or so - then do both knees up together and hold as long as you are comfortable. This is called the "tuck".

2) Now, stretch your lower back system. Stick left foot across your right leg and under right knee while lying on right side, and twist torso to roll shoulders flat on bed, holding for 20-30 seconds - do same on other side. Caution: If you have lower back degeneration, lower back pain, etc., don't do this side-torsion stretching exercise. *Alternatively, this will be more forgiving and not so strenuous: Keeping drawn-up knees together, with your back staying flat on the bed (or floor) roll the knees from side to side as far as you can, and "holding" each side a second or two. A minimum of 15 rolls.*

3) Do "roll-ups" for the abdominal muscles (abs) - lying flat on your back with knees drawn upward (do not do this exercise with your legs extended because it unduly strains the lower back) and hands locked behind the head if that is comfortable, do multiple sit-ups ("crunches"). While doing roll-ups, strive to raise your shoulders off the bed or floor - without raising just your head which would only exercise your neck. An attractive alternate is the "jack-knife", in which you raise knees toward chest simultaneously with each sit-up. If you do enough abs, you'll be proud and happy to expose your flat tummy at the beach next summer.

4) Stand next to bed (for a soft landing in case you fall backward) and do plenty of "deep knee bends". Standing erect, start your "squatting" by doing 10 reps with slight knee-bending for warm-ups, then another 10 (do all you can) deeper, etc. until you are doing max depth of "squat" and your bottom is hitting the bed. If you feel no leg stress, or very little stress, squat deeper. Hold something heavy if you can. This is a very important leg exercise, because you are strengthening muscles that enable you to push your body up to standing position when arising from a chair, etc., and that facilitate your seating yourself easily when going in the other direction.

5) Next, sit on edge of your bed or other high seat. With knees together grab edge with both hands and sit up straight while raising knees as high as possible, up and down. Work up to 25 reps - or more if you can.

6) Same, but with legs spread as far apart as you can. Brings different gut strap-muscles into play.

7) Stand with back firmly pushed against a wall (at door jamb or other place where you can grab something if needed for support) and push your arms high, all the way up, alternatively right and left. This stretching exercise will keep your upper back muscles happy, which is very important if we don't want to walk bent forward, and when we stand erect.

8) Stay right there and now finish up this easy-but-effective routine, by doing up to 25 stiff-leg kick-raises (high as possible) with each leg. Caution: Do not raise both legs at the same time. Hee, hee!

If you can do push-ups (lie on tummy and push yourself up with hands on floor until your arms are fully extended, keeping your body stiff and straight) do them as your final move. As many as you can, for it strengthens the upper arms. Even a little helps.

Last and best - walk quickly into the kitchen and get your cup of coffee. Then sit, sip and feel good about yourself. You've earned it.

Your doctor will provide an exercise regimen if you ask. Or, go online where you will find several websites that detail special exercises for Parkinson's patients *("Parkinson's Disease - Fitness Counts", "The Center For Neurologic Study"*, etc). Search for *"Parkinson's Exercises"* or *"Movement Disorder Exercises"* and you'll find dozens and dozens of exercises.

However, your doctor may refer you to a Physical Therapy office, where trained PT practitioners will put you through practical moves and probably will give you a page or two (complete with pictures) of exercises to do at home. PT practitioners can be of important help to MD people, especially for stretching exercises designed to loosen muscles that are tight and inflexible. Do these and you'll walk better.

Also of value are Recreational Exercises such as Swimming, Biking, Hiking and Dancing (Square-Dancing Club?). Even some regular daily activities have an aerobic, or conditioning benefit: Household chores such as mopping and vacuuming, walking the dog, gardening and yard work.

A program of regular exercise performed 3 or more times every week can strengthen the heart and lungs, improve stamina and endurance, reduce stress, improve mood and combat depression, and help control high blood pressure, high cholesterol and diabetes. There's enough there to excite even the most stolid types!

Non-powered-wheelchair folk (I've seen quite a few in my gym, working with weights) aren't left out for they can derive good cardio exertion on arms, legs and torso with sustained powering of their vehicles. If the gym doesn't excite you, perhaps you can consider acquiring bicycle-type or other workout equipment that is readily available for purchase at Sears and many other retail stores. They are not expensive and take up very little space at home. Some even can be folded and pushed under a bed (wake up the cat first). "Armchair

Aerobics" exercise videos can be found at sporting goods stores or video areas of department stores.

Stretching exercises should be done every day with each exercise being done at least 3 times for 3 to 5 in-and-out breath counts (or as specified by your doctor), and you can do them anytime throughout the day (while watching TV, for example). Choose a time when you are well-rested and your medications are working.

Many of us do not breathe deeply. We should try to keep in mind inhaling fully with each breath, for shallow breathing can adversely affect our quality of speech and lead to tension and fatigue. A good breathing exercise asks that you stand tall and with feet hip-width apart, cross arms over one shoulder, take in a deep breath and begin lifting arms up and open, breathe out and lower your arms to starting pose. Repeat 5 or more times, with DEEP breaths.

NEGLECT EXERCISING

AT YOUR PERIL

12 – DIET AND NUTRITION

The information in this chapter is derived from research and other sources of readily-available material, and is repeated for reference, only.

The prevailing wisdom concerning nutrition for most MD patients is nothing much more than common sense. Eat a balanced diet including all food groups and consume sufficient calories to maintain your weight (what you normally did before onset of your affliction to maintain energy and general health). Of course, one should observe the usual caveats about too much fat, too much red meat, etc. Sufficient fiber and fluids (gospel tells us to drink 8 eight-ounce glasses of *filtered and purified* water each day - avoid drinking tap water.) should be taken to avoid constipation.

Also recommended is taking Calcium (at least 500 mg) in combination with Vitamin D in sufficient quantity (400 mg) to prevent osteoporosis.

Side-note regarding time to take medications: There are clinical findings about Sinemet (80% of we ParkinPeople are prescribed that medication) that should be made part of our knowledge: Sinemet should be taken 15 to 30 minutes before meals to ensure the most predictable absorption (the same for Sinemet CR, although it is not thought as critical for the absorption). If the drug produces nausea, a light, low protein snack should be taken with it before meals, or if that doesn't work take Sinemet with meals. Also, if this medication causes too much diskinesia (involuntary movement), that condition may be improved by only taking it <u>with meals</u>. You should discuss this with your physician.

13 - MEDICATIONS AND TREATMENTS

Movement Disorder treatment includes medications that may include Anti-epileptics, Anti-seizure medications, Beta-Blockers, Dopamine Agonists, Tranquilizers and others. There is some duplication in medications for different MDs. All of this sort of information must originate with your physician, with the following provided only for reference.

The medication most commonly prescribed for PARKINSON'S DISEASE ("PD") is Sinemet, a combination of levodopa and carbidopa (the latter delays the conversion of levodopa to dopamine until it reaches the brain, often lessening or even preventing levodopa side effects). The brand name Sinemet is proprietary and not a generic term referring to just any carbidopa/levodopa formulation, for other names that can be prescribed include Atamet and Sinemet ER, which can be considered equivalent to Sinemet. *Generic formulations of many medications are available at lower cost.*

Carbidopa/levodopa (Sinemet, et al) and the dopamine agonists (listed below) are the most effective medications for treatment of PD, with carbidopa/levodopa being considered the most effective medicine to control tremor, rigidity and bradykinesia (slowness of movement).

A "Controlled Release" form of Sinemet is available as Sinemet CR, for use by prescription in the event a patient has too-rapid "wearing off" by immediate-release Sinemet. It is absorbed more slowly and allows longer dopamine activity in the brain. Ask your physician about this.

Dopamine patches are expected to be on the market soon, pending FDA approval. These are applied to the skin on the shoulder or back and worn for 24 hours before being replaced by a new patch.

Another class of medication used for Parkinson's and other MDs is known as *dopamine agonists*, which have a similar chemical structure to dopamine and treat in similar manner. They provide symptomatic benefit as "monotherapy" (are taken *without additional* medication) in early disease and as adjuncts to levodopa in later disease. They all have significantly longer "half-lives" (refers to the time it takes for a drug to be broken down in the body) than levodopa. Your doctor no doubt will want to make you aware of these dopamine agonist drugs:

Bromocryptine
Pergolide
Ropinirole (Requip* - see below))
Pramipexole (Mirapex**- see below)
Cabergoline
Apomorphine

Parkinson's experts are <u>enthusiastic</u> about three new drugs the FDA approved in 1997: Mirapex and Requip (trade-names), both of which are approved for use alone or with levodopa drugs. Combining one of these two new medications with levodopa drugs permitted advanced patients to reduce these doses up to 25% for Mirapex and up to 31% for Requip.

Also recently approved by the FDA is Tasmar (trade-name), which also may be taken with levodopa drugs. In trials, patients with a stable response to levodopa drugs who took Tasmar experienced significant improvements in daily activities such as talking, walking and dressing.

Also on the market are: Parlodel, Permax, Amantadine, Selegiline and Eldepryl.

HUNTINGTON'S DISEASE treatment focuses on reducing symptoms, preventing complications and providing support and assistance to the patient. Physicians often prescribe various medications to help control HT emotional and movement problems:

Antipsychotics
Antidepressants
Tranquilizers
Mood-Stabilizers
Botulinum toxin

DYSTONIA. Several medications are being used in the treatment of DYSTONIA, including Sinemet, which was mentioned above for Parkinson's. Also of help to Dystonia patients are BOTOX injections, as is the Deep Brain Stimulation detailed later. Oral medications are useful in treatment of this disease, as well as complimentary care such as Physical Therapy and Speech Therapy.

TOURETTE'S SYNDROME: Drug therapy may include anti-anxiety medications, or certain anti-psychotic dopamine receptor antagonist drugs. Again, injections of Botulinum Toxin may be prescribed.

STROKE victims may be benefited by oral medications, as directed by the physician, but rehabilitation is highly important, administered by Physical Therapy (PT), Speech Therapy and Occupational Therapy. We all may benefit by observing the following measures that may help prevent Stroke:

Do not smoke
Exercise regularly
Limit dietary intake of salt, alcohol and saturated fat.
Maintain body weight within an ideal range
Use airbags, seatbelts and child safety seats in automobiles
Wear protective helmets when engaging in contact sports, horseback or bicycle riding.

TREMOR (Essential Tremor) often does not require treatment, and lifestyle changes such as those listed immediately above may improve symptoms, but severe essential tremor can be reduced using medications in most cases. Medications include many of those already listed for other MDs, plus

Beta blockers
Benzodiazeines
Carbonic anhydrase inhibitors
BOTOX injections also may be used

ATAXIA involves clumsiness, or loss of coordination, which may affect the fingers and hands, the arms or legs, the body, speech or eye movements. It is a symptom, rather than a specific disease or diagnosis. Ataxia may be caused by a number of different medical or neurologic conditions, and it is for this reason a person with such symptoms must seek medical attention to determine the underlying cause, and to get appropriate treatment. Severity varies widely as does the progress of this condition.

Treatments include medications as prescribed by a doctor, speech therapy also may help with swallowing difficulties, and physio-therapy.

HEREDITARY ATAXIAS are a group of genetic disorders characterized by slowly progressive in-coordination of gait, and often is associated with poor coordination of hands, speech and eye movements.

EPILEPSY is a neurologic condition that affects the nervous system. Also know as a *seizure disorder.* The seizures in this condition may be related to a brain injury or a family tendency, but most of the time the cause is unknown. Its diagnosis can cause the patient unusually traumatic attitude malaise, and usually is made after the person has had at least two seizures that were not related to a known medical condition such as alcohol withdrawal or extremely low blood sugar, but the cause is unknown for about half of its victims.

There are dozens of medications used in treatment of Epilepsy, and individualized surgery is an alternative for people who do not respond to medications. For full information, go to the *www.epilepsy.com* website, where a resource library is prominent.

In my opinion, there is hope for MD relief right now rather than sometime in the future. It is a promising new therapy called I.V. (intravenous) Glutathione to help slow the process of nerve cell degeneration.

Glutathione is found in all cells of the body, being a powerful naturally-occurring brain-protecting anti-oxidant playing a substantial role in the functioning of the body's immune system and the recycling of vitamins C and E after they have been oxidized. It is significantly decreased in PD patients (and in Autism, cancer, HIV, Diabetes, Alzheimer's, cardiovascular, pulmonary and liver diseases, and others), with the deficiency occurring in the portion of the brain in which the dopamine-generating neurons are concentrated. It is an important antioxidant that functions as a scavenger of free radicals, detoxifies heavy metals and toxic chemicals, just for starts.

The effects of I.V. Glutathione treatment on Parkinson's Disease patients are reported to be immediate and dramatic, and often alleviating the depression that so often accompanies Movement

Disorders and similar diseases. This treatment reportedly is very safe and without significant side effects. Initial treatments can begin several years after onset of the disease, and are administered by simple injection at home (if qualified), in a doctor's office or during a treatment course lasting several days in a clinic.

One doctor reports 80% of his Parkinson's patients trying I.V. Glutathione have dramatically positive results from this treatment, and of those who had this treatment 80% remain on it a year after starting, and continue to improve. A study done in Italy reported a month of twice-daily applications of I.V. Glutathione improved all patients and showed a 42% overall decline in disability that lasted two to four months after the therapy was stopped.

Wellness Health and Pharmacy is a <u>compounding</u> pharmacy, and is the sole provider of their patented Glutathione of enhanced stability that will not degenerate by oxidizing, as will others. Incidentally, for personal application Wellness Health will supply their IV Glutathione with the syringes, needles, prep pads, etc. If you are going to have the IV done by your doctor, why not consider the possibility of saving money by placing an order to be shipped to your doctor's office, and be charged only for the I.V. there).

In addition to their stable IV Glutathione, Wellness Health has an <u>*oral*</u> liposomal Glutathione that can be mixed with water or juice of choice (I can report from personal experience there is no noticeable taste induced by this liquid). As an added convenience, Wellness Glutathione is available in the following forms: nebulized, nasal spray, suppositories, transdermal (topical) and sublingual troches.

We can arrange to have literature mailed to us with a phone call, and can purchase (very reasonably) from their extensive list of hypo-allergenic health aids (example: Neuropathic and Arthritic Pain Management, for both topical and injection application) direct from Wellness Health, 3401 Independence Drive, Suite 231, Birmingham, AL 35209.
(800) 227-2627 [T: (205) 879-6551]
e-mail: *mail@wellnesshealth.com*
www.wellnesshealth.com

Scientifically-controlled studies are being conducted on an ongoing basis, on this promising treatment. Perhaps this treatment may be used in lieu of L-dopa, which we are warned sometimes may cause liver damage and itself contribute to the generation of free radicals that worsen Parkinson's in the long run.

It has been mentioned previously, but we should know about BOTOX (Brand name for Botulinum Toxin, Type A), a naturally-occurring substance that has been in use since about 1990 for relief of DYSTONIA (involuntary rhythmic contractions of the muscles). Today, most of BOTOX use is for facial and similar cosmetic improvement, but some specialists use it for PD tremors and other such applications. It is injected into muscle that is contracting abnormally, with the usual result of partially weakening the nerve to the muscle for about four to six months, and has proven very useful in people who suffer from abnormal muscle contractions.

BOTOX injection is a medical procedure, and often is guided by an electro-myogram (EMG). The hollow-needle EMG locates the area of worst contraction within the muscle, allowing the BOTOX to be injected at the site that will produce the best result, which is to prevent unwanted muscle contractions. It may result in weakness of the muscle treated, and its benefits will diminish and fully wear off in four to six months. Thus, for long-term illnesses, the injections must be repeated if you wish its benefits to continue.

If you have excessive muscle spasms such as hand and arm tremor, you should consult with your neurologist (who may refer you to a specialist) about having BOTOX applied to the offending muscle(s).

Side effects usually are transient and mild-to-moderate in nature other than loss of strength in muscle involved. Best check with your doctor regarding possible interactions with medications being taken. The procedure is not inexpensive, so perhaps you should check with your HMO or other health insurance provider, first. For further BOTOX information call the manufacturer: 1-800-530-6680.

A new treatment, APOKYN, has been approved in 2004 by the FDA and now is available for use in "off" periods if needed. It is a prescription injectable medication that is used "as needed" to treat loss of control of movement disorders. It is injected just under the skin and not into a vein. It is used in addition to other medications, not instead of them. For information, ask your doctor or call 1-877-727-6596. Online: *www.apokyn.com.*

PHYSICAL THERAPY also should be dealt with in this category, but has been discussed in the chapter "*Alternative and Complimentary Therapies*", so I'll not go into detail here. Sufficient to say PT can be greatly supportive of your goal directed toward physical and mental progress. The experts who assist and train you are highly educated and able, and will encourage your every effort. They're good people.

A little-recognized item of interest is a mind-boosting product called "Advanced Ginkgo Smart" a formulation of natural nutrients and herbs. Ginkgo Biloba has long been thought to boost the smarts.

The September, 2004, issue of AARP Bulletin carried some information that may be helpful in the future. Up to 50,000 Medicare beneficiaries were to get coverage for some of the costliest life-saving prescription drugs under a demonstration program that was to run until the drug benefit starts in 2006. Co-payments were to be the same as required by the drug benefit, but only a small fraction of the overall cost.

The $500 million demo applied to those who enrolled by September 30, 2004. For info on possible other such programs, call (866) 563-5386. or go online to:

www.medicare.gov
<http://www.medicare.gov>.

You really should have a compact pill container, such as the one that has a row of seven little "boxes" with a snap lid on each. Take it with you - everywhere.

Another item that may bring you a feeling of security is a "Medic-Alert Bracelet", or equivalent, that can bring medical assistance in a hurry if needed.

14 - SURGERY

Activa Tremor Control Therapy

The FDA recently approved an important tool for controlling tremors: *The Activa Tremor Control Therapy,* which consists of the surgically implantation of a wire deep within the brain and connected to a pulse generator, similar to a cardiac pacemaker, implanted near the collar-bone. Whenever a tremor begins, the patient can activate the device merely by passing a hand-held magnet over the generator.

This system (device) delivers a mild electrical stimulation that blocks the dysfunctional brain signals that cause tremor. Effects often are dramatic.

Pallidotomy

Similar to Thalamotomy (see below) except the lesion is placed in a different part of the brain, and is by far the most commonly performed lesioning surgery.

Data suggests patients may benefit from this procedure with reduction in tremor, rigidity, bradykinesia and "off-time" by 15 to 50 percent at four months, and even up to four years after surgery. Some patients with tremor were shown to have a reduction of up to 75 percent.

Pallidotomy procedure has proven to be quite helpful especially to patients in the late stages of Parkinson's.

Thalamotomy

This procedure involves using a heat-sensitive probe to create a small lesion in the thalamus of the brain, and is very effective at reducing tremor as well as essential tremor in PD, by as much as 90 percent. Long-term benefits lasting up to 10 years have been reported.

Thalamotomy as a surgical procedure destroys a specific group of cells in the thalamus, and is aimed at 5 - 10% of those with disabling tremor in hand or arm. It is very effective.

Deep Brain Stimulation

DBS is a relatively new technique involving placement of a metal electrode into the brain. The electrode is continuously stimulating the brain with a high-frequency. The DBS results in a marked reduction of tremor in 92 percent of PD patients, with results lasting up to 8 years or more. However, similar to thalamotomy, the other motor symptoms of MDs are not greatly reduced.

Gamma Knife Radiosurgery

Similar to the previously discussed surgeries thalamotomy and pallidotomy, in which a small lesion is created in the brain by means of an external beam of radiation rather than by physical surgery. The safety of this procedure and its long-term benefits are not known.

Oddly, one type of surgery (i.e. DBS) can be done on one side of the brain and another (pallidotomy or thalamotomy) on the other side, with satisfactory results for the patient.

There are a number of promising treatments still on the horizon, for which practitioners have much hope.

15 - ALTERNATIVE AND COMPLIMENTARY THERAPIES

Traditional Chinese Medicine

This is a complete system of medicine that originated thousands of years ago in China. TCM treatments include diet, exercises such as t'ai chi and the Qi Gong breathing, herbal preparations, acupuncture, acupressure massage, physical therapy and moxibustion. The latter involves the use of heat at specific energy points on the body - either applied directly or to the acupuncture needles - as a way to add energy.

Acupuncture is the best-known of the Chinese treatments, with some of the benefits being relief of pain, improvement of fatigue, strengthening of the immune system, ridding the body of toxins, and reducing muscle spasms and tremor.

Acupuncture has been well studied and proven to be effective for a variety of problems. It is applied by medically-certified practitioners, perhaps with a combination of acupuncture and Chinese herbal formulas. MDs can be controlled and their progression slowed, but not completely cured. The sooner the treatment is started after onset of the MD, the better the outcome.

Ayurvedic Medicine

AM has been the traditional medicine in India for more than 5,000 years, and perhaps is the oldest medical system in existence. It is based on the premise the body naturally seeks harmony and balance. In Ayurveda, proper balancing is accomplished through food and diet, herbs, meditation and breathing, massage and yoga poses.

Ancient Ayurvedic texts provided a description of Parkinson's Disease, and described a successful treatment using a substance known as *Mucuna pruriens,* a twinelike plant native to India. Medically significant amounts of Levodopa have been isolated from the beans of this plant, and research shows PD patients who took *Mucuna pruriens* had improvement of almost one entire stage in the 1-5 Hoehn and Yahr staging system.

Herbal Medicine

Going back to ancient times, there always has been an understanding of the power of plants and plant products as medicine (many of today's most powerful and effective drugs actually come from plants and herbs). According to the World Health Organization, some 4 billion people, or 80 percent of the world's population, use some form of herbal medicine.

It is becoming increasingly popular in the West, and herbal teas, supplements, extracts and tinctures are enjoying a resurgence.

In the United States, herbal medicine practitioners may be physicians, osteopaths, naturopaths, nutritionists, or more traditional "herbalists".

Homeopathy

Homeopathy is widely practiced in the U.S. and throughout the world. The basic idea is you can stimulate the body's own healing mechanisms to fight illness by administering a homeopathic remedy that would cause similar symptoms in a healthy person ("like cures like").

- Some of the many remedies that would be recommended for MD people treat: Trembling and tremor of head and hands.
- Trembling, droopy eyelids, staggering, weakness and fatigue.
- Trembling hands and excessive salivation.
- Stiff but trembling or twitching limbs, with itchy back and spine.
- Twitching, restlessness, and jealous or suspicious moods.
- Mild tremors and stiffness that lessens with movement.

Relaxation, meditation and stress reduction

There are many types of mind-body therapy, everything from prayer to yoga to counseling to dance to breathing exercises, to touch just a few. Some of the approaches that fall into this broad category include biofeedback, guided imagery, hypnosis, transcendental meditation, psychotherapy, spiritual healing, music therapy, art therapy, breathing exercises, humor therapy and other forms of relaxation.

Prominent in this broad category are support groups, for participation by MD people provides an outlet for anxiety and stress, plus the added benefit of sometimes yielding education and information otherwise difficult to attain.

Psychotherapy or counseling can help calm down your overall emotional state, allowing more energy for healing and fostering more positive thoughts and actions, which in turn speeds recovery.

Biofeedback is a treatment method using monitoring instruments that provide you with various physical information such as pulse, body temperature and other indicators of stress which you don't normally monitor. By wearing a biofeedback monitor you learn to adjust your thinking to then control bodily processes such as blood pressure, temperature, gastrointestinal functioning and brain wave activity. These are not normally under your direct control physically.

Creative therapies such as dance, music or art therapy use the creative arts to address health concerns. Studies have shown music therapy to have a beneficial effect on the emotional functions, activities of daily living and general quality of life of MD patients.

One benefit to the creative process is it seems to tap into a different pathway to the brain for MD folk, many of whom find their symptoms lessen, or even disappear when they are involved in a creative act. (Perhaps the brain says: "Out of sight, out of mind").

Writing and journaling are other effective mind-body therapies - they offer the benefit provided by the positive power of writing.

Prayer and mental healing techniques usually describe an altered state of consciousness due to a spiritual experience, or the "flow of energy" or healing via another person's hands. Studies have shown these techniques to be effective, especially concerning stress and energy-related problems.

Meditation techniques are most common in Asia and are an integral part of Buddhism, Hinduism, many other Asian religions and yoga. Regular meditation or guided relaxation and imagery have notable effects on blood pressure, anxiety, chronic pain, body tension and immune response and can clinically reduce cortisol levels (a measure of the body's stress level).

Guided imagery can be an effective technique for healing. You can use your own imagery or follow a book, audiotape or practitioner. If you are feeling stress, you might envision progressively relaxing each part of your body as you relax on a sunny beach, or envision the body's healing capabilities focusing on an organ or process that isn't working as optimally as possible.

To try a simple guided imagery exercise, close your eyes, take several deep breaths and focus on a particularly bothering symptom. Prompt an image to appear representing your symptom, accept and study it, then tell the image how you feel about it, aloud or to yourself, and visualize its replying and telling you why it's there and what it wants. Talk to this image, asking if it will let your problem abate and continue the dialogue until you arrive at some sort of agreement with the image.

Relaxation and Breathing Exercises can lead you to a "place I enjoy going to", choosing a real place. Experience your being there vividly through your memory of it, and relax while you relish your re-living a good experience at this place you love, with closed eyes and deep breathing while concentrating wholly on this enjoyable experience. A few minutes of this sort of excursion can return you to "now" with relief from the pain or stress condition(s) from which you wanted to escape. Relaxed.

Laughter Therapy

A good howl will reverse a bad anything!

Laughter is very important to our well-being and general health, for it can lessen pain while increasing pleasure and inducing a feeling of happiness. We all know for a fact that folks who are good-humored and laugh often (really *laugh*) are much more likely to be healthy and stay healthy.

The reasons are obvious. Watching a good comedy movie or TV program takes us away from the present and onto that cloud of lightness floating up there where happiness lives. A funny book will do the same. Can you, no, *will you*, make a list of all the fun things, places, people, movies, books, games, etc., etc. that you can conjure up in your now-lightened mind? Which do you want to pursue? Which *will* you engage in?

When your list is finished (for the time being until you think of more fun stuff), wouldn't it be expressly helpful to contact a person you really like, or love, and tell him/her of your delightful excursion into humor and invite that beautiful person to join you and laugh and laugh away all our problems?

Physical Therapy

We all know what this therapy is: PT is a science. A science involving not just knowledge of all the moving parts of our bodies but of the effective mental component that is the natural companion of physical improvement.

Perhaps your doctor will have prescribed it as an important element in your successful treatment (Always keep in mind this fact: *All treatments are blessings, and all will be successful, and all will detach you from being negative to being a positive and lovably interesting you).*

PT is *physical* and it is good and beneficial *therapy*, for it not only involves but requires your voluntary and forceful participation in elevating muscle firming, endurance, generally increased mobility and fitness level, and strengthening of targeted body parts, while advancing your overall physical endurance and mental attitude. Again, one's mind cannot function well if the body is not in good condition. That happy state is entirely achievable even though one may be affected by a MD. Just ask a PT instructor!

Why not look into the mirror and ask the same of yourself? See how good you look while nodding.

The many variations of PT will provide a very complete basis for your interesting workouts, and (with your willing participation) will promote better posture, balance and control of bodily movement, while reducing stiffness and rigidity (which can be reduced dramatically by specific stretching exercises). Now, that may sound like "too much", but you can make it all happen.

Manual Healing, Bodywork and Energy Work

There are many different types of massage and manual healing, but they can be of good benefit to ParkinPeople. What they have in common is use of a practitioner's hands and touch to promote healing and well-being. Here are just a few of them.

Massage

Can be very beneficial for MD people due to its ability to achieve relief for muscle and joint pain, stiffness and stressfulness while inducing that wonderful plateau of euphoria and sense of relaxed well-being. There are several types of massage, each with its own variations and methods of application. Take your choice. The masseuse(s) will explain the merits of each, which may include sleep improvement, for example. [You should be aware of and (hopefully) avoid those establishments offering more, sometimes much more, than a simple massage! Whee!].

Acupressure

Also known as "pressure point massage". Can help MD People having symptoms of nausea, excessive salivation, muscular pain and rigidity, and anxiety, not to mention decrease of anxiety and fatigue symptoms. This sometimes is thought of as being a companion of acupuncture and has been around for a long, long time.

Cranial Massage

Also called Craniosacral Massage, delivering a light touch and Acupressure on the cranium (also called "noggin"), to alleviate MD-induced tension and encourage increase of energy. Who doesn't like a good head rub? Ask your doggie about this.

Osteopathic Manipulation

There is clear evidence and research to support the application of this therapy. It treats the patient who has musculoskeletal spasm, aches and pains caused by misalignment of the body's structure (the bony part) in order to re-establish normal skeletal alignment and return usual function of treated elements. Osteopathy also can deal with symptoms or underlying causes of distress, and be very helpful in returning the patient to normal functioning, overall.

Reiki

The central thrust of Reiki is the tapping into a universal "energy force" by the practitioner and then passing that "healing energy" into the patient, who will receive it where most needed in mind or body. Practitioners will either touch the patient or merely pass hands over the body, with resulting benefit being realized by the patient in proportion to that person's level of acceptance of the treatment. Thought to relieve both physical and emotional suffering.

Exercise

An essential component of successful therapy, and considered a therapy complimentary to clinically-directed assistance. It will improve muscle and joint strength, and maximize physical ability while preventing further degeneration and disability resulting from illness or injury. It will increase bone density. Exercise is discussed in detail earlier in this book, so further description will be found there.

Yoga and T'ai Chi

Both emphasize gentle stretching and balance-oriented exercises, of value to MD people due to their deliberate movements done with patient concentration. They may deliver to MD patients an improvement in mood and corresponding decrease in depression. Yoga is ancient in origin and use, and deals with combining harmony and balance within the body, mind and spirit (with the universe), when applied by physical and breathing exercises coupled with meditational techniques.

Traditional medicine has found many applications for Yoga among its many forms that feature improvement in muscular distress, poor balance, depression, breathing difficulty (lung function), carpal tunnel syndrome, sleep disorders, tremors, joint misfunction and flexibility, to name just a few. T'ai Chi has similar benefits, and also can be practiced at home.

Naturopathy

Naturopathic Medicine is the science of identifying and treating *causes* of illness rather than *symptoms*, and calls upon many disciplines for its assets, among which are included: Acupuncture, Homeopathy, Herbal Medicine, Dietary and Nutritional Medicine, Manipulation, Massage and other beneficial applications. Its defined intent is to achieve a good balance of physical, emotional, mental and spiritual constituents, all of which assist the body's natural ability *to heal itself.*

Acceptance Of The Right Therapies

With input from your doctor, you must determine if you wish to, or need to reconcile your traditional treatment with one or more alternative treatments, then select which "medicine(s)" you will at least try, as being the one or ones most applicable to your specific needs.

16 - SAVE ON DRUGS

Although it is not widely publicized, pharmaceutical companies have programs to help people who can't afford their prescriptions. You can get information on these programs by contacting:

1) GlaxoSmithKline - "Orange Card Program" to assist low-income seniors - (888) 672-6436.
2) Pfizer "Living Share Card" - (800) 717-6005.
3) Pfizer "Sharing The Care Program" - (800) 984-1500.
4) Parke-Davis/Pfizer "Connection To Care Program" - (800) 707-8990
5) To redeem a 20-40% discount on 200 medications (including Sinemet, Sinemet CR, Comtan, Parlodel and Requip made by any of the following: Nevartis, Astra Zaneca, Abbott, Aventis, Orthomcneil Janssen Pharmaceuticals or GlaxoSmithKline), join the *"Together Rx"* prescription saving program. Call (800) 865-7211.
6) The Pharmaceutical Research and Manufacturers of America - call (800) 762-4636 hotline and ask for the Directory of Prescription Drug Patient Assistance Program (over 1,400 medicines offered free).

The California legislature has passed a bill approving CA residents' buying medications from Canada. You should find out if your state approves this issue, for it could save you tons of money.

Furthermore, your doctor may have information concerning low-cost medicines, or sources that will deliver them free or at a fraction of US retail prices.

17 NUTRITIONAL AND HERBAL "SUPPLEMENTS"

There are quite a few commonly-used vitamins, minerals and herbal preparations that may be of help to MD People.

As the term "supplement" suggests, the items listed below should not be substituted for, but may be added to your usual and necessary foods specified by your physician such as fresh vegetables and fruits, grains, proteins, poultry, fish, red meat, dairy products, and so forth.

All reputable vendors of supplements carry a variety of *multivitamins*, so one may have a choice for the one most appealing and suitable. As the name implies, these preparations combine an extensive assortment of vitamins, minerals and other nutritional elements. The strong advice of the author is to buy your supplements from a source that sells *natural* preparations, rather than those that are artificially produced. Your doctor surely will agree.

Anti-oxidants are effective in combating the health-threatening effects of those nasty free radicals. They include vitamins C and E (in combination), and *alpha lipoic acid*, an anti-oxidant said to be especially effective against free radicals that functions to materially boost the effectiveness of other anti-oxidants. I strongly suggest you discuss this anti-oxidant with your doctor, for it may affect the life-spans of Glutathione and Coenzyme Q-10, both of which are of significance to us.

Selenium falls into this classification, also, and is claimed to boost circulation, plus protection of nerve cells. An anti-oxidant of importance is *Coenzyme Q-10* (it is frequently referred to as *CoQ10*) and will be recommended by many doctors as being necessary (mine surely did!).

Vitamin D, because it very materially effects the good and proper assimilation of *Calcium,* which we know to be essential in maintenance of bone density and health. When selecting Calcium products, find one that includes Vitamin D, which is necessary for Calcium to be effectively utilized.

B and B-Complex vitamins - considered by many to be necessary to good health, with Vitamin B-6 included in a B-Complex preparation. Your doctor should be willing to discuss this class of essential vitamins at length so you will be comfortable with them. Ask for his recommendation regarding the B vitamins you should take.

Calcium is important, and is noted above as being a companion to Vitamin D, for together they act to strengthen skeletal elements, not to mention maintenance of muscular health. The usual daily minimum of Calcium is 1,000 mg.

Joint-maintenance formulations are said not only to help maintain, but actually build cartilage, and usually include *Glucosamine, Chondroitin, MSM* and other joint-support factors

Magnesium also works to benefit a healthy nervous system, and may help to alleviate rigidity as well as muscular cramps. And, it's dirt cheap.

Ginkgo Biloba has been shown to sharpen short and long-term memory, and can support anti-oxidant activity in the brain, eyes and the entire cardio system. GB should be discussed with your doctor, since its effect can be beneficial to MD patients.

There are dozens and dozens of supplements on the market, each of which affects some aspect of health, and which can confuse people who have not studied this field or who are not being guided by those qualified in this direction. A full list here would be non-productive and confusing so this discussion of supplements will end here.

18 - COUNSELING

Psychologists and social workers can be an important part of our healthcare team. Adjustment to a diagnosis of MD often is distressful, and sometimes prolonged.

But over time people get past the feeling of being overwhelmed by this diagnosis, and begin planning how to accommodate the reality of MD in their lives. Short-term counseling with a capable psychotherapist can be immensely helpful during this period.

If you experience mood changes such as depression and anxiety (not to mention anger) for more than two weeks, ask your physician to refer you to a competent therapist. He also may prescribe an anti-depressant that can be taken safely with MD drugs.

19 - DRIVING

For most people driving represents independence, freedom, control and competence, and is necessary for our everyday happiness. For many people, being able to drive is important economically, for they depend on this ability to get to and from work

It is a complex skill. Our ability to drive safely can be affected by changes in our physical, emotional and mental condition, all of which can be brought about by a MD.

Most importantly, the effects of this disease can materially slow our *reaction time.*

You should be able to continue driving in the early stages of the disease, and you are taking medications that control the symptoms. If you stay fit and active physically, you should be able to drive safely, but if there is doubt about your driving capability, you may benefit by being referred to a center or specialist who can give you off-road tests to determine how MD is affecting your ability to drive. He may also offer training to improve your motor skills while your affliction still permits you to drive safely.

At the time we are told (and honestly realize) we no longer can drive safely without endangering ourselves and others, it comes as a severe jolt, for we are losing the independence of driving ourselves. But all is not lost, for with planning we can get to the places and people we want to see. Consider:

- Rides with family and friends
- Taxi cabs
- Shuttle vans or buses for seniors
- Religious and other local transportation conveniences
- Public transportation (especially those systems maintained for people with physical or mental deficiencies - they actually may pick you up at your residence)
- Walking

Call ElderCare facilities for information on transportation.

CAUTION! If you have *any* doubt about your ability to drive with a fully alert mind (medications can make you feel light-headed, or worse) or if your reaction time may be getting pretty slow, please do as I have: Stop driving entirely before something bad happens. It's tough, but you may save a life.

20 - PERSONAL THOUGHTS

Sometimes it's difficult to be optimistic, and even more troubling to be cheerful, but we can and must adopt a hopeful outlook and live to enjoy each day of life to its fullest because it won't be here tomorrow. Life is a gift to be treasured.

Life doesn't owe us anything. It's *what we are giving life* that matters.

There is wonderful substance and true beauty in the following writing by Irma Bombeck, who had an unusually optimistic way of looking at and living life, and whose writings for years brought laughter and good feeling to millions of people. However, when she learned she soon would be taken by cancer, she set down her deepest thoughts about her life and the way she should have lived certain parts of it.

Here they are (you may need a hanky, for she'll get you right where you live):

I would have gone to bed when I was sick instead
of pretending the earth would go into a
holding pattern if I weren't there for the day.
I would have burned the pink candle sculpted like a
rose before it melted in storage.
I would have talked less and listened more.
I would have invited friends over to dinner even if
the carpet was stained, or the sofa faded.
I would have eaten the popcorn in the 'good' living
room and worried much less about the dirt

when someone wanted to light a fire in the fireplace.

I would have taken the time to listen to my grandfather ramble about his youth.

I would have shared more of the responsibility carried by my husband.

I would never have insisted the car windows be rolled up on a summer day because my hair had just been teased and sprayed.

I would have sat on the lawn with my grass stains.

I would have cried and laughed less while watching television and more while watching life.

I would never have bought anything just because it was practical, wouldn't show soil, or was guaranteed to last a lifetime.

Instead of wishing away nine months of pregnancy I'd have cherished every moment and realized that the wonderment growing inside me was the only chance in life anyone ever gets to assist God in a miracle.

When my kids kissed me impetuously, I would never have said, "Later. Now go get washed up for dinner."

There would have been more "I love you's". More "I'm sorry's".

But mostly, given another shot at life, I would seize every minute, look at it and really see it, live it and never give it back.

Stop sweating the small stuff.

Don't worry about who doesn't like you, who has more, or who's doing what.

Instead, let's cherish the relationships we have

with those who do love us.

Lets think about what God HAS blessed us with, and what we are doing each day to promote ourselves mentally, physically, emotionally, as well.

We have one shot at this and then it's gone.

I hope you all have a blessed day.

21 - WHAT WILL BE OUR LEGACY?

"I have fought a good fight. I have finished my course. I have kept the faith"
- Holy Bible *(II Timothy 4:7)*

Regardless of the future outcome, we will have won, *really* **won**, when we know we have given Life our very best shot.

We cannot ask more of ourselves! We take comfort and pride when seeing in the mirror the reflection of a *winner*, a person who drew upon inner resources to ride over a perceived obstacle and press ahead with dedication and courage to personal achievement. We see a person who has realized and put into perspective the *hopeful prophecy* of this book:

ALWAYS
Be thankful for the years we've already been given.
Accept our condition in good grace.
Look ahead with positive determination to make our future one of true accomplishment.

No matter who we are, what we have accomplished, and without regard to our condition, we all must contemplate not only how we live from day to day, but how we will be remembered when we respond to The Beckoning Of The Final Voice.

I speak of the "Legacy Of Life", the manner in which those who knew and survive us remember our "persona"- the true person who lived in our heart and assuredly was reflected so faithfully in our daily living.

We, as do all other living things, have a life-span during which that legacy grows, is constituted and established. At the observance or our passing, such as a memorial or any similar event, many of those who knew us during our brief stay on this planet will be in attendance, and will envision us standing in full view, naked of all earthly trappings for The Final Human Judgment Day. We will be perceived honestly, exactly as these people knew us, good, bad or indifferent.

We are taught there is an "Afterlife", into which those who are judged worthy will ascend, and into which those who fail to qualify will descend. We mortals are not given the ability, the right, to see into this future aspect of "being", and must hope for the best and live accordingly. But, there is another Afterlife, a creation of "being" we are enabled to bring to those who knew us during Life.

It is absolutely true that we will continue to exist, *to live*, in Memory, and will be brought to mind from time to time by those who knew us, for the rest of their lives. In what did we excel? What did we accomplish? *What place did we <u>earn</u> in_their hearts?*

This Afterlife is a legacy! A legacy filtered through experience, and accrued only to those who knew us, and who always will view us only as they did during our earthly existence. If we strove to overcome our burden and in so doing brought joy and happiness into the lives of those we loved, their legacy from us will brighten the eye, lighten the load and bring spring into the step.

Even though we may be ill with a Movement Disorder, no matter its effect upon us, it's our call during Life to share the good that comes to us, and be helpful to and considerate of others. We will be judged accordingly.

A legacy involving money or other earthly goods is transient and will diminish and be lost. And forgotten. However, we have within us the ultimate capability to bequeath to our loved ones a permanent legacy, the Ultimate Legacy beyond value that transcends all others and will live for all time.

It is the special beauty of the inner self that dwells in the heart and is given without condition to another. This very special legacy lives in a beauty beyond reckoning. That legacy is Love.

Plant a flower.